BREATHE

A Guide to Managing Anxiety in a Turbulent World

Barbara Sheen

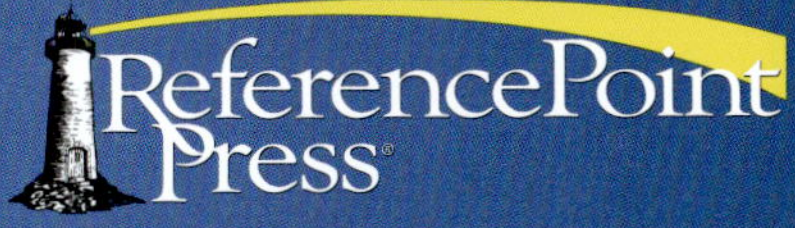

San Diego, CA

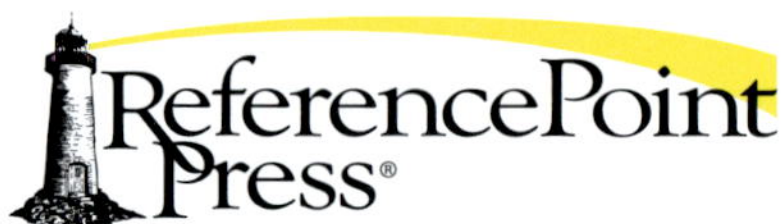

Printed in the United States

For more information, contact:
ReferencePoint Press, Inc.
PO Box 27779
San Diego, CA 92198
www.ReferencePointPress.com

LIBRARY OF CONGRESS CATALOGING-IN-PUBLICATION DATA

Names: Sheen, Barbara, author
Title: Breathe: A Guide to Managing Anxiety in a Turbulent World/by Barbara Sheen
Description: San Diego, CA : ReferencePoint Press, Inc., 2025. |
Includes bibliographical references and index.
Identifiers: LCCN 2024044665 (print) | ISBN 9781678210069
(library binding) | ISBN 9781678210076 (ebook)
Subjects: LCSH: Anxiety disorders--Juvenile literature. | Anxiety disorders--Treatment--Juvenile literature.

CONTENTS

Living in Turbulent Times

Daneisha Carter is a young woman who had her first panic attack when she was eighteen years old. Although the incident badly frightened her, she thought it was an isolated occurrence and tried to forget it happened. Nevertheless, the attack was just the beginning of her struggle with anxiety. As she recalls:

> After that incident I noticed I wasn't myself. I started waking up feeling weird. I didn't know how to explain it to anyone. . . . In certain situations, like car rides I would get super anxious, grabbing on the door handle because I was fearful something was going to happen to me. April 2022, I was at a fair with my cousin and brother, there was a shootout. I have never been so scared in my life. It definitely amped up my anxiety. As time went on, it felt like my anxiety was getting worse and worse. I became very stressed out. I started losing focus on school, work, everyday tasks, and I had personal issues at home I was battling. My health even started to decline. Everything was happening all at once and I couldn't control it. . . . Wishing that all this pain could go away. I even became suicidal multiple times but never acted on it.[1]

Unable to dismiss what was happening, Carter took a variety of steps to regain control of her life. Although she still deals with anxious moments, she has learned how to manage them. Anxiety no longer consumes her life.

A Worldwide Mental Health Crisis

Carter is one of approximately 301 million people worldwide who struggle with debilitating anxiety. According to the World Health Organization, anxiety is the most common mental health condition in the world. Although anxiety levels peaked during the height of the COVID-19 pandemic, issues with anxiety have not gone away since. In fact, in 2021 US surgeon general Vivek Murthy declared that the United States was experiencing a mental health crisis. This crisis is ongoing. ComPsych Corporation, a provider of mental health services, reports that nearly one-quarter of Americans who sought mental health treatment through their employers in 2023 did so due to anxiety.

It is not just workers who are troubled by anxiety. Anxiety is a common emotion that arises due to overwhelming stress. It causes worry and fear related to future and past events, as well as physical symptoms. Although it can affect anyone—no matter a person's gender, age, or race—some groups are more likely to develop debilitating anxiety. Females are one of these groups, with the US Department of Health and Human Services reporting that women are twice as likely as men to have an anxiety disorder. Adolescents are also disproportionately impacted. A 2024 research study conducted at Children's Hospital Colorado found that problems with anxiety among Colorado youth ages eleven to sixteen had nearly doubled since 2018. Young adults ages eighteen to thirty and members of the LBGTQ community are also disproportionately impacted. So are individuals who have experienced poverty, violence, or trauma in their lives. National Basketball Association forward Marcus Morris is one of these individuals. He grew up in a Philadelphia neighborhood besieged by gang violence. He maintains that the trauma and violence he dealt with in his youth led to his developing problems with anxiety and depression as an adult. He recalls, "I've seen guys get shot just for sitting on the wrong front step. You wake up every day thinking, 'How am I going to protect myself?'"[2]

Why Now?

There are many issues driving the current mental health crisis. Twenty-first-century life is stressful. We are constantly beset by minor and major stressors. Long lines, traffic jams, malfunctioning electronics, and looming deadlines are just a few of the minor stressors that plague us. Add in other concerns related to family, relationships, health, finances, work, and school, and stress can quickly become overwhelming. Plus, there is the constant stream of grim news and graphic images on news feeds, on social me-

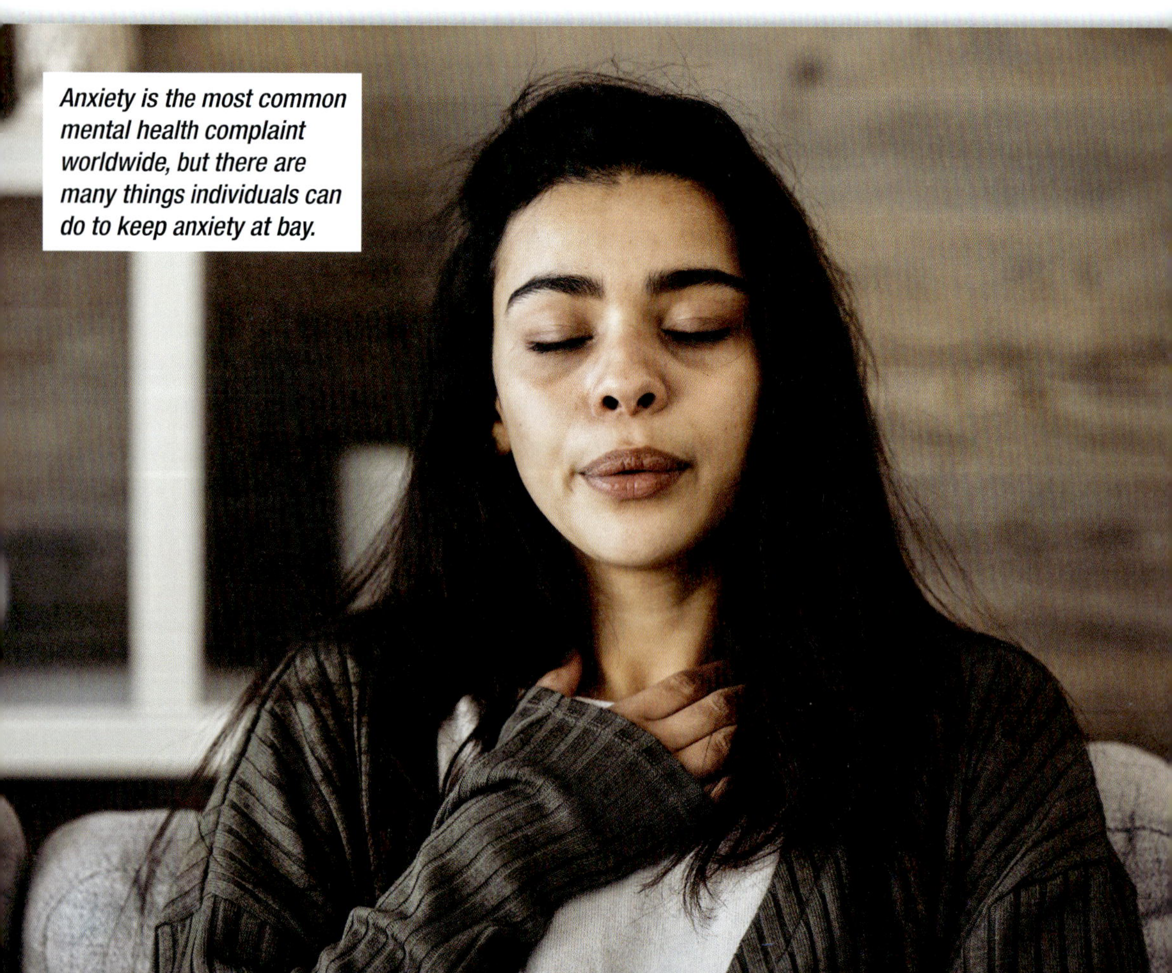

Anxiety is the most common mental health complaint worldwide, but there are many things individuals can do to keep anxiety at bay.

dia, and in broadcast and print media. News about global crises such as racism, gun violence, wars, and climate change create fear and uncertainty about the future, which can cause or heighten anxiety symptoms. As youth mental health advocate and social impact strategist Jorge Alvarez explains:

"In recent months I've been experiencing anxiety at the thought of our current climate crisis. . . . I get anxious at the thought of what the state of the world will be or even feel like 10 years from now."[3]

—Jorge Alvarez, youth mental health advocate

> Learning about the severity of climate change has made me a bit more worrisome and anxious at times. When I struggled with my mental health, it felt like yet another issue that was out of my control and as though "doomsday" was inevitable. . . . In recent months I've been experiencing anxiety at the thought of our current climate crisis. . . . As a recent college graduate, I already have a lot of important life decisions to make. But add the fact that the planet may not be alive in another 50 years and all these decisions feel pointless. I get anxious at the thought of what the state of the world will be or even feel like 10 years from now.[3]

Taking Control

Clearly, stressors that cause anxiety are everywhere. It is impossible for people to keep stress out of their lives. And based on all that is going on in the world today, it is likely that the future will present more anxiety-provoking challenges. Nonetheless, there are many steps individuals can take to keep stress and anxiety at bay. Doing so can help you cope during these turbulent times and prepare you to handle future trials more easily. As Carter advises, "Keep fighting because there is going to be light at the end of the tunnel."[4]

"Keep fighting because there is going to be light at the end of the tunnel."[4]

—Daneisha Carter, anxiety sufferer

CHAPTER ONE

Understanding Anxiety

On the surface, award-winning actor Jonah Hill appears to be a carefree person, but he has been badly affected by debilitating anxiety for many years. To gain more knowledge about his condition, in 2022 Hill wrote, directed, and starred in *Stutz*, a documentary film that explores his battle with anxiety and features discussions about the condition with renowned Los Angeles mental health therapist Dr. Phil Stutz. Making the film helped Hill understand anxiety, his personal triggers, and how to manage the condition better. He explains, "Through this journey of self-discovery within the film, I have come to the understanding that I have spent nearly 20 years experiencing anxiety attacks, which are exacerbated by media appearances and public facing events."[5]

Based on this newfound understanding, Hill stopped participating in these events. He also made other changes in his life to help improve his mental health. Although he is not cured, he is doing much better. He hopes that the film will inspire other anxiety sufferers to learn about the condition so they, too, can take actions toward managing it.

Anxiety Starts with Stress

Severe anxiety like Hill's is caused by overwhelming stress. Stress is a physiological reaction to challenging, frightening, or unpredictable situations that are difficult to cope with and that the brain perceives as a threat. Such threats are known as stressors or triggers. Stressors may be severe, moderate, or mild. They may be real or imaginary. Severe stressors are usually traumatic events such as experiencing a violent assault or the death of a loved one, among other things. Moderate and mild stressors are typically common occurrences like meeting a deadline, fighting traffic, or performing in a competition; while imaginary stressors are unreal situations that people create in their minds. Even happy events that cause uncertainty about the future, such as starting a new job or getting married, can be a trigger, as can remembering a past stressful event or seeing stressful images. But no matter the trigger, the brain's reaction is the same. Upon perceiving a threat, it activates a primitive physiological reaction known as the fight-or-flight response. Anxiety—which is a feeling of fear, nervousness, dread, and worry—is part of this reaction.

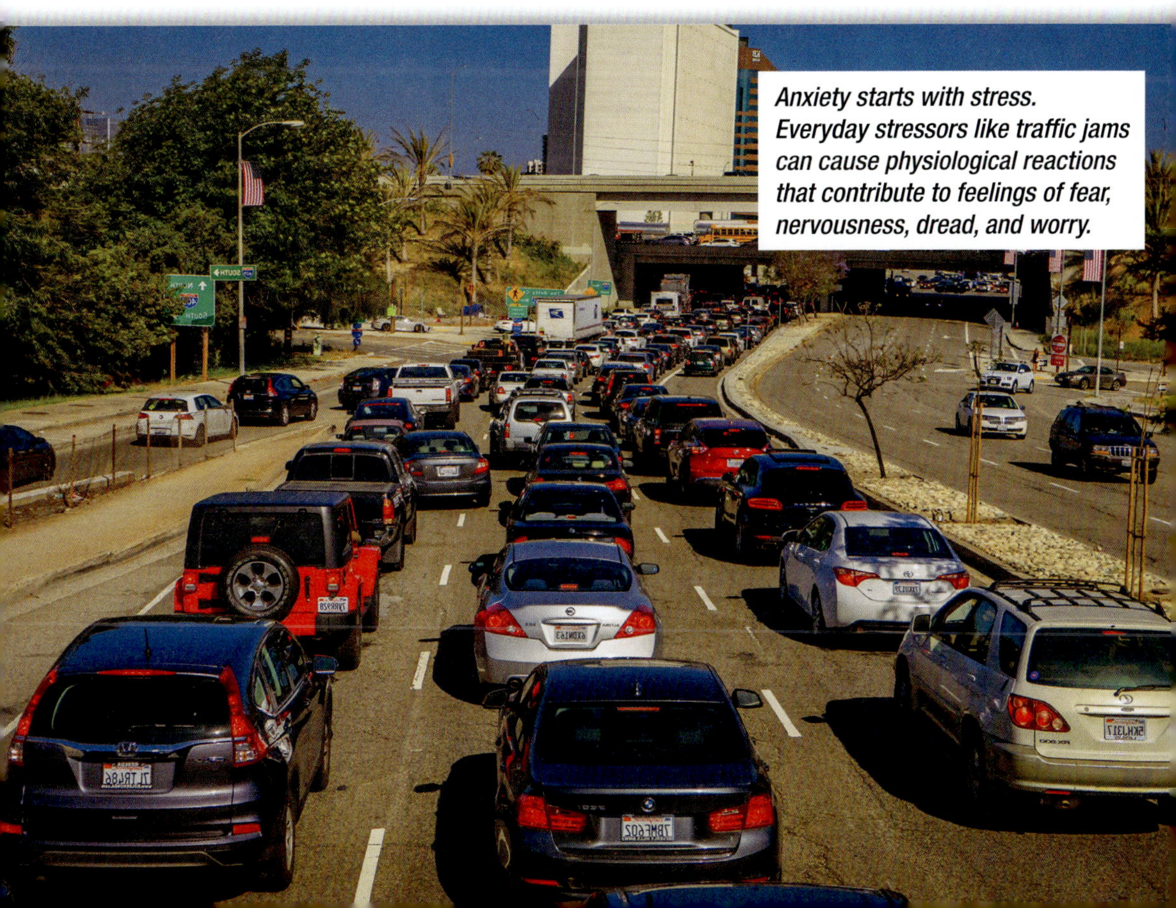

Anxiety starts with stress. Everyday stressors like traffic jams can cause physiological reactions that contribute to feelings of fear, nervousness, dread, and worry.

An Overreaction

The fight-or-flight response begins in the amygdala, a part of the brain that regulates fear and other emotions. When the amygdala perceives a threat, it signals a part of the nervous system called the sympathetic nervous system to prepare the body to fight or flee. In response to this signal, cortisol, adrenaline, and other stress hormones flood the body. Their presence sets off a chain reaction that supercharges the body. As a result, blood pressure, heart rate, breathing rate, and blood sugar levels rise. Muscles tense, digestion slows, and the pupils dilate, among other symptoms. While this reaction gives you extra energy, improved vision, reduced perception of pain, and more power to defend yourself, it also causes your heart to pound, your stomach to feel upset, and your body to tremble, sweat, and feel jittery. And as stress hormones course through the brain, they make you feel anxious, irritable, confused, and unable to focus on anything besides the stressor.

The fight-or-flight response protected early humans from physical harm, but it is an overreaction to most modern stressors. As Simoné Sanders, a Texas marriage and family therapist, explains, "Our amygdala, or emotion center of the brain, is similar to a smoke detector, in that it can't tell the difference between real or perceived danger. Whether you burn your food or your house is on fire, the smoke detector goes off either way."[6]

"Our amygdala, or emotion center of the brain, is similar to a smoke detector, in that it can't tell the difference between real or perceived danger. Whether you burn your food or your house is on fire, the smoke detector goes off either way."[6]

—Simoné Sanders, marriage and family therapist

When Anxiety Becomes a Chronic Problem

The fight-or-flight response is usually temporary. Once an alleged threat has passed, the body calms down and stress and anxiety symptoms dissipate. For instance, runners often feel anxious

A Boiling Pot

Chronic anxiety and anxiety disorders are often misunderstood. In an article on the National Alliance on Mental Illness website, the organization's communications manager, Luna Greenstein, describes what having an anxiety disorder can feel like:

> Imagine your mind as a typical four-burner stove top. At all times, there's a small pot at a rolling boil on the back burner. That's Anxiety. Every possible thing you could ever be anxious about is floating around in this pot, churning all day long. Depending on what happens throughout the day, a thought can pop up out of the pot and intrude your thinking—"Oh God . . . did I lock the front door?" Then it goes back down—"Yes, of course." Then other thoughts pop up—"Why did my boss give me that look the other day?" "Am I saying the right things?" "Do I look okay?" "Do I smell bad?" The churn is constant.
>
> If something goes wrong, the churn worsens. And the small pot might even be replaced with a medium-sized pot. More water. More pressure. More thoughts. On days when Anxiety is severe, a large pot will slam onto a front burner—your anxious thoughts taking center stage on the forefront of your mind.

Luna Greenstein, "The Difference Between a Disorder and a Feeling," National Alliance on Mental Illness, October 10, 2019. www.nami.org.

before a big race, but once the race is over and the stressor is gone, their bodies relax. However, if you are overwhelmed by persistent stress or multiple stressors, your fight-or-flight response does not turn off. Therefore, the body does not get a chance to calm down and recuperate. Instead, stress hormones continue to stream through your body, keeping you in a hypervigilant state. This makes you feel even more stressed and anxious and can cause you to develop chronic anxiety.

Chronic anxiety is not a minor issue. It can, and frequently does, disrupt a person's life. Unlike mild, short-lived feelings of anxiety, chronic anxiety can stick around for years. It causes the same physical symptoms as stress and short-term anxiety. Plus, it causes you to feel fidgety and nervous almost all the time. In addition, chronic anxiety causes a host of persistent mental symptoms. These include unrelenting, distorted thoughts and feelings of extreme fear and worry, even if there is no factual evidence to justify these fears.

Even when these fears have some basis, they are typically out of proportion to the real situation. Individuals with chronic anxiety tend to imagine the worst. For example, if a family member is late getting home, chronic anxiety can make you believe that your loved one has been killed or maimed in a fiery accident when it is more likely that your family member got caught in traffic or stopped at a store to pick up a few things. Or if you are going on a first date, anxious thoughts and fears can convince you that you will say and do all the wrong things, making you a social outcast who will never be loved.

Indeed, fears created by chronic anxiety can upend your life. They can make you doubt yourself and your sanity, thereby lowering your self-esteem and causing you to constantly seek out the reassurance of others. They can also cause you to isolate yourself and keep you from trying new things. This is how Danielle E., a young woman who has battled chronic anxiety for years, describes her experience:

> Instead of hanging out with friends, having fun, or even being able to study and focus on school, my days were spent worrying about one thing after another. Fears that I was going to die, fears that I had a brain tumor, fears that I was going blind, fears that I had diabetes, fears that I would be kidnapped, fears that my house would burn down, fears of people, fears that I wasn't good enough, pretty enough or I wasn't smart enough, fears of failure and fears that I had no future. . . . These fears have been crippling me all my life. They have made me distance myself from having friendships, relationships, jobs, school, social events and anything that could trigger these fears more and that could cause me more anxiety. My fear of failure and of people has resulted in me skipping many days of school and to make many excuses to friends to not hang out or go to social events.[7]

Chronic Anxiety and Health

Not only can chronic anxiety lower your quality of life, if it is not controlled, it can take a toll on your general health and well-being. Insomnia, as an example, is a common health issue for individuals with chronic anxiety. Being constantly worried and on edge makes it hard to fall or stay asleep. Lack of sleep can negatively affect your memory, mood, and concentration. It also can weaken your immune system, increasing your risk of catching colds and developing infections. Making matters worse, anxiety puts a strain on your digestive system and your heart. People with chronic anxiety often struggle with irritable bowel syndrome and acid reflux, among other digestive issues. Some develop an eating disorder. Moreover, chronic anxiety has been linked to high blood pressure and poor heart health.

Chronic anxiety is also associated with inflammation. Although inflammation is the body's way to heal itself, excessive or chronic inflammation damages healthy cells. Not surprisingly, it is associated with the development of several physical and mental health

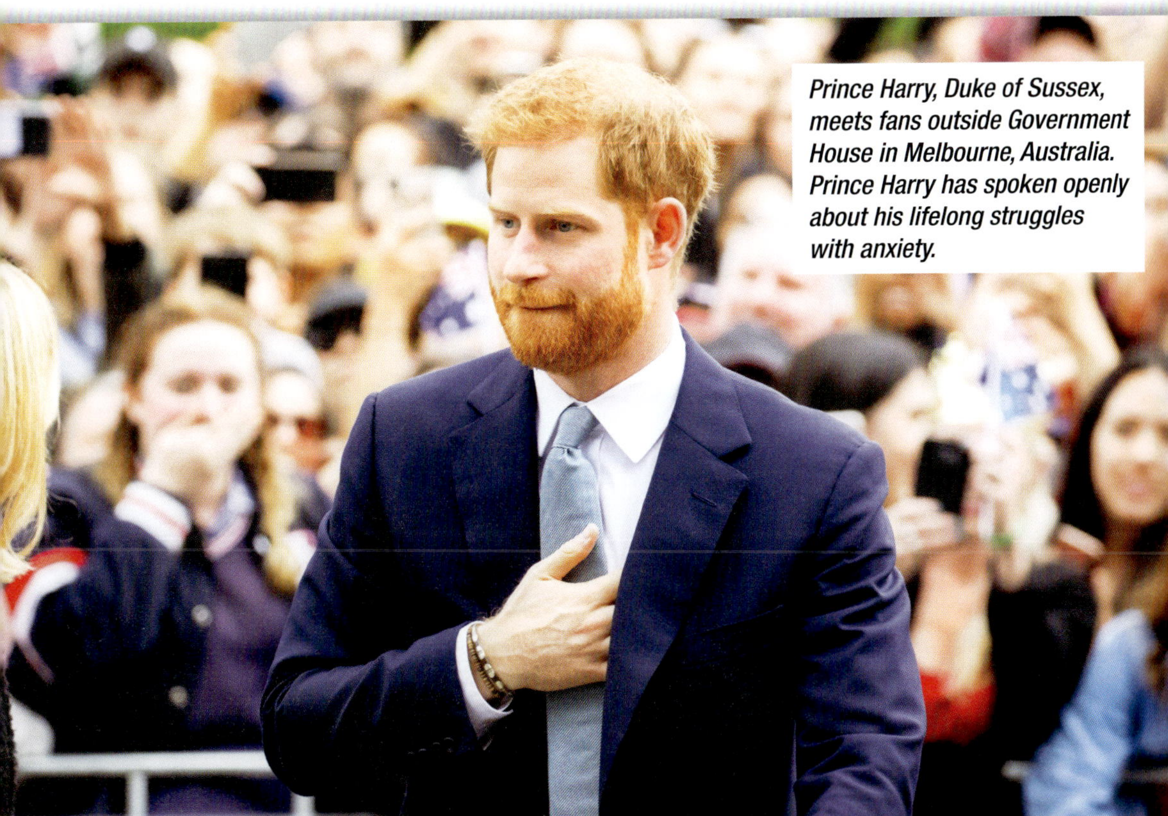

Prince Harry, Duke of Sussex, meets fans outside Government House in Melbourne, Australia. Prince Harry has spoken openly about his lifelong struggles with anxiety.

problems, including cancer, diabetes, anxiety, and depression. Indeed, chronic anxiety can be so hard on the mind and body that some individuals self-medicate with drugs and alcohol in an attempt to calm themselves. This not only causes other health problems, it also worsens anxiety. Prince Harry, Duke of Sussex, as an example, has struggled with anxiety since he was a child. His condition spiraled out of control when his mother, Princess Diana, was killed in a car crash. He tried to cope by using drugs and alcohol. These actions not only did not help him, they also raised his anxiety. He recalls, "I was willing to drink, I was willing to take drugs, I was willing to try and do the things that made me feel less like I was feeling. I would probably drink a week's worth in one day on a Friday or a Saturday night."[8]

Chronic anxiety may also be involved in the development of an anxiety disorder. Anxiety disorders are mental illnesses that cause intense, relentless anxiety along with symptoms specific to each disorder. They include phobias, social anxiety disorder, generalized anxiety disorder, and panic disorders. Social anxiety disorder, generalized anxiety disorder, and panic disorders

Laughter Helps Relieve Stress and Anxiety

"Laughter," an old saying proclaims, "is the best medicine." Indeed, studies have shown that laughter has many physical and mental health benefits. Laughter inhibits the production of stress hormones and stimulates the release of endorphins. Endorphins are feel-good chemicals that reduce pain and improve mood. Laughter also improves circulation, oxygen intake, and muscle relaxation, activities that can lessen the physical symptoms of anxiety. In addition, focusing on humorous subjects counteracts negative thoughts.

Although it may be difficult to find things to laugh about in turbulent times, there are strategies to help bring more laughter into your life. They include spending time with upbeat people with whom you share jokes and funny stories. Watching funny movies, TV shows, and YouTube videos rather than sad or upsetting ones is also helpful. So is keeping a humor journal in which you record at least one thing that made you chuckle each day. Similarly, posting jokes, comic strips, and silly photos and sayings in a spot where you can see them is a good way to promote laughter.

are among the most common. Social anxiety disorder is characterized by fear and worry related to any social situation, while generalized anxiety disorder causes excessive, irrational worry and dread about almost everything. Panic disorder causes recurrent panic attacks. These are sudden attacks of extreme fear, which come on without warning and which frequently mimic a heart attack. During a panic attack, it is not uncommon for people to feel like they are about to die. Toronto Blue Jays first baseman Joey Votto for example, admits that panic attacks have sent him to the hospital on several occasions. He says that during these attacks he was convinced that he was dying.

"I was willing to drink, I was willing to take drugs, I was willing to try and do the things that made me feel less like I was feeling."[8]

—Prince Harry, Duke of Sussex

Recording Thoughts and Feelings

The mental and physical health issues, combined with the negative thoughts and fears that characterize chronic anxiety, can make you feel like anxiety has taken control of your life and will never go away. Nonetheless, anxiety can be tamed. Practicing a variety of self-help strategies can produce relief. Keeping an anxiety journal is one strategy that has proved to be helpful. In this journal, you write about the thoughts, situations, people, and physical symptoms that precede and accompany your anxious thoughts and feelings. Rating the intensity of the anxiety and what you did to get relief is also often part of this process. Mental health experts say that keeping an anxiety journal can help you gain insight into specific triggers and thought patterns that provoke or raise your anxiety, so that you can take steps to manage them. In addition, putting your negative thoughts and feelings down on paper can make them seem less frightening. It allows you to take a step back and separate your troubling thoughts from yourself. And it helps you clear these thoughts out of your mind, which calms you, improves your mood, and helps you focus on more positive things. Moreover, rather than keeping your anxious thoughts bottled up inside you, which can lead to depression, a journal gives you a safe, nonjudgmental place to vent. In fact, a 2021 Dartmouth College study found that when college students recorded their thoughts through this type of journaling, they reported feeling less anxiety and depression.

Another variety of journaling known as happiness or gratitude journaling also is valuable in reducing anxiety. As the name implies, this type of journaling involves recording at least one thing (and hopefully more) that makes you happy or that you are grateful for each day. Several studies suggest that doing so helps people shift out of an anxious mindset to focus on happiness and the good

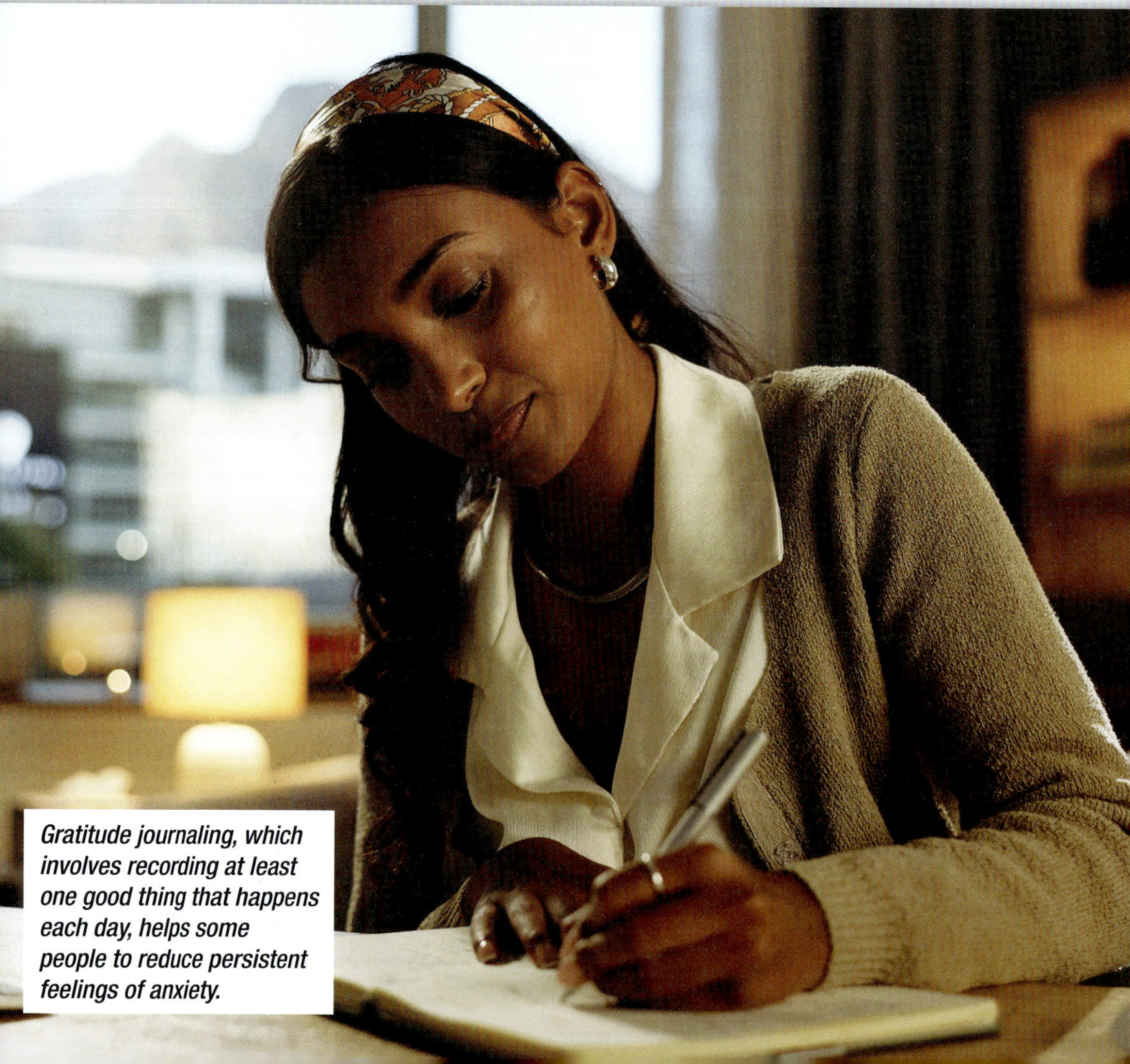

Gratitude journaling, which involves recording at least one good thing that happens each day, helps some people to reduce persistent feelings of anxiety.

in the world, which is especially valuable during turbulent times. As a matter of fact, feeling and expressing gratitude puts the brakes on the fight-or-flight response. It reduces the release of stress hormones, while stimulating the release of dopamine and serotonin, feel-good chemicals that make you feel calm and contented. As University of Virginia psychologist Jessica Stern explains:

"Daily gratitude practice can help alleviate stress and calm negative emotions. One way this works is by shifting our attention."[9]

—Jessica Stern, University of Virginia psychologist

> Daily gratitude practice can help alleviate stress and calm negative emotions. One way this works is by shifting our attention. Rather than ruminating about something we regret saying, rehearsing a conversation in our head, focusing on what we wish we could have, or worrying about work the next day, gratitude focuses the mind on the "glimmers," good thoughts that can reorient us to positive feelings of connection, abundance, and good fortune.[9]

An added benefit of any type of journaling is how easy it is. It does not require a set structure. You can journal on paper or digitally. If you do not know what to write about, some journals and apps feature prompts to help you get started. And if writing is not your thing, your journal can consist of voice or video recordings. Or it can take the form of lists, doodles, or illustrations. The important thing is getting into the habit of journaling regularly. Many individuals find that journaling at a set time helps make it part of their daily routine.

Challenging Anxiety-Provoking Thoughts

Once you have identified the situations or fears that trigger your anxiety, the next step is tackling them with solutions. Challenging anxiety-provoking thoughts by examining them logically and questioning and evaluating their validity can help you develop a new way of thinking. This is not as difficult as it sounds. Say, for instance, going for an annual checkup triggers your anxiety. Since anxiety causes your thoughts to immediately jump to the worse possible scenario, you might worry that you will be diagnosed with a dreadful disease that will cause you great pain and suffering and end in your premature death, even though you are feeling fine.

The first step in challenging such thoughts is to assess how valid these thoughts and the consequences they predict are. Think about whether you have had these thoughts before other checkups and whether your dire predictions have ever come true. Consider how many times you have been diagnosed with a serious health issue in the past and, if a problem was discovered, whether the outcome was as catastrophic as you imagined. Answering these questions should help dispute the validity of your negative thoughts.

Next, defy your false thoughts by imaging alternative possibilities. Instead of dwelling on sickness and death, think about how strong you are and envision a positive or, at the very least, neutral outcome. Remind yourself that you are generally healthy, and even if you had health issues in the past, you were strong enough to overcome them. They did not ruin your life. Finally, try to come up with possible solutions to ensure your anxiety-provoking thoughts do not come true. In this situation that might include taking steps to boost your health, such as eating healthy foods, getting plenty of sleep and exercise, and avoiding risky behaviors. Undertaking these steps can help you identify thinking errors, take negative thoughts less seriously, and develop more flexible thinking. As a consequence, you should find it easier to manage anxiety.

Mastering Relaxation Techniques

As the winner of five gold medals and one silver medal, track cyclist Laura Kenny (formerly Laura Trott) is Great Britian's most successful female Olympian in history. Kenny, who is the first British female athlete to win gold medals in three Olympics, was bestowed the title of dame (which is the equivalent of knighthood) by Queen Elizabeth II for her achievements. But her success has not always come easily. Like many athletes, Kenny deals with anxiety before a competition, a problem which is also known as sports or performance anxiety. To calm down so that she can perform at her best, she practices controlled deep breathing before going out on the track. "It sounds stupid," she admits, "but by thinking about your breathing, it stops you thinking about anything else. If you push your belly out when you take a breath in, like doing the opposite to what you think you should do, it really helps."[10]

"It sounds stupid, but by thinking about your breathing, it stops you thinking about anything else."[10]

—Laura Kenny, British Olympic gold medalist

Inhale Calm, Exhale Anxiety

Like Kenny, many elite athletes practice controlled deep breathing to deal with pre-competition anxiety. When people are anxious, they tend to breathe rapidly and shallowly up in the chest. Their shoulders rise a little, but their stomach does not move in

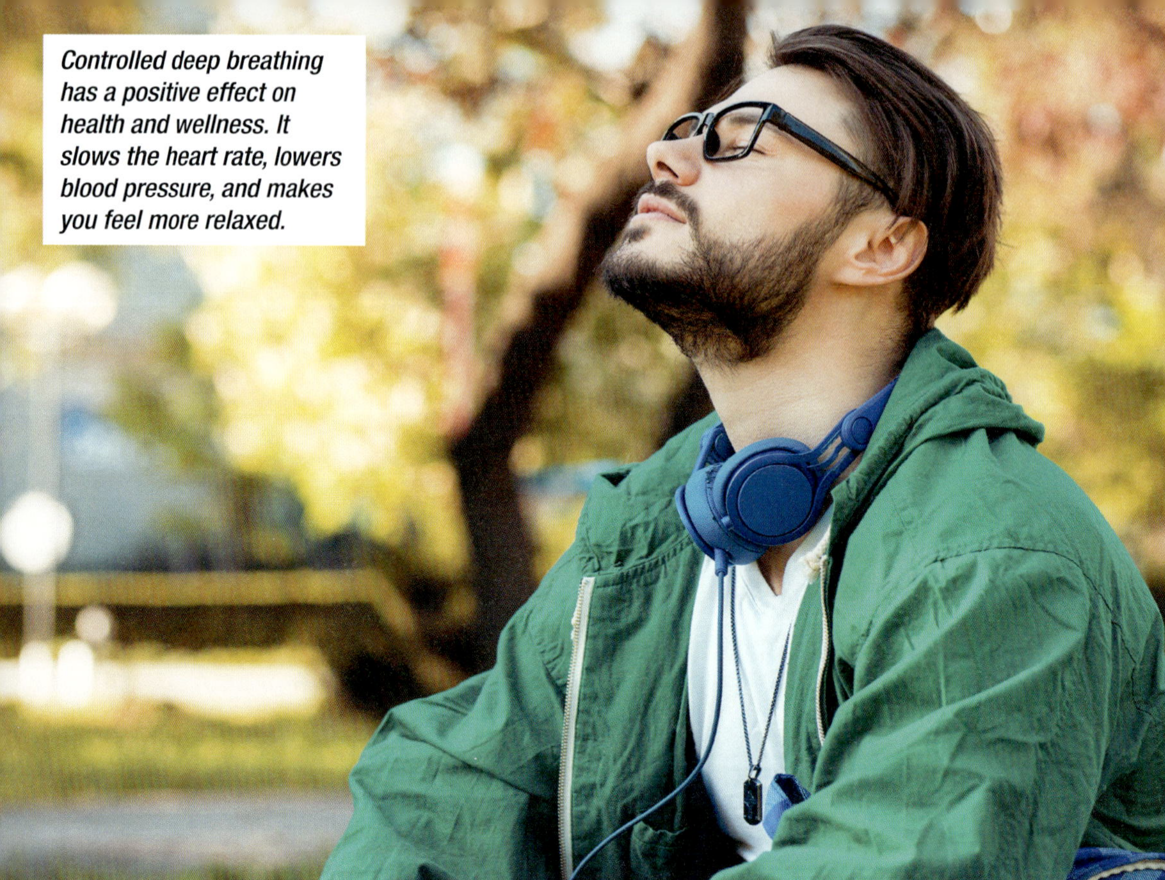

Controlled deep breathing has a positive effect on health and wellness. It slows the heart rate, lowers blood pressure, and makes you feel more relaxed.

and out the way it should. Fast shallow breathing prevents enough oxygen from getting into the lungs and enough carbon dioxide from getting out. As a result, individuals tend to feel breathless, tense, irritable, disoriented, and panicky, which intensifies the fight-or-flight response.

In contrast, when people are calm and relaxed, their breathing is slow, deep, and regular. They breathe from their diaphragm, a muscle that runs between the chest and abdomen, and their stomach moves out and in. Slow, deep breathing increases the flow of oxygen throughout the body and lets excess carbon dioxide escape. In the process, it creates a feeling of calm by activating a relaxation response. This response triggers the release of feel-good chemicals that counteract the fight-or-flight response. Even yawning deeply appears to have a calming effect on the nervous system, since it brings more air into the lungs. Speed skater and eight-time Olympic medalist Apolo Ohno says he yawns repeatedly before a race. “It makes me feel better. It gets the oxygen in and the nerves out,”[11] he explains.

Numerous studies indicate that controlled deep breathing has a positive effect on health and wellness. It slows the heart rate, lowers blood pressure, and makes you feel more relaxed. It can help thwart a panic attack and is a simple and easy way to tamp down anxious feelings. Plus, it can be practiced anywhere at any time, while you are sitting, standing, or lying down. There are many deep breathing exercises. Most start with breathing in through the nose for a count of three to five, then out through the mouth for the same count, repeating this process until you feel calmer. This is akin to inhaling the aroma of a steaming bowl of soup, then blowing on the soup to cool it down. Sigh breathing is a variation of this method. It involves inhaling deeply through the nose, pausing for three counts, then exhaling very slowly, as if you are giving a long, drawn-out sigh. And to help increase calm feelings, as you inhale you might try visualizing an ocean wave rolling in. As you exhale, envision the wave rolling out with your anxiety. Silently repeating a calming word or phrase as you breathe deeply can also increase calm feelings, especially if you sync the rhythm of your breathing to the word or phrase. And to check that you are breathing from your diaphragm, you can put your hands on your abdomen as you breathe in, feeling it expand as you inhale and contract as you exhale.

Making deep breathing exercises a daily practice is ideal. Practicing controlled deep breathing regularly helps your body learn a new pattern, which can help you manage anxious feelings when they arise. But even taking a few deep breaths before facing a challenging situation can reduce anxiety. To help you get started, there are many free apps and online videos.

Meditation

Meditation is another useful tool in combating anxiety’s physical and emotional symptoms. In fact, a 2022 study published in *JAMA Psychiatry* indicates that daily meditation practice is as

Progressive Muscle Relaxation

Progressive muscle relaxation is another technique that helps manage anxiety. The fight-or-flight response causes muscle tension. Prolonged muscle tension is a common symptom of chronic anxiety. Prolonged muscle tension can cause muscle pain and cramps, which exacerbates anxiety. Progressive muscle relaxation is a way to relax tense muscles, thereby reducing physical discomfort as well as anxiety. Progressive muscle relaxation involves tensing various muscles and muscle groups one at a time as you inhale, then relaxing these same muscles as you exhale. To get started, lie on your back, close your eyes, and take a few deep breaths. Then starting with your feet, curl or tense your toes for a few seconds. Then uncurl your toes, focusing your attention on how relaxed your toes feel. Continue this procedure, working your way up your body from your feet to your legs, buttocks, chest, shoulders, hands and fingers, neck, jaw, cheeks, and eyes. Once you are finished, lie still for a few minutes and breathe deeply and slowly, thinking only about how good your body feels.

effective as a daily dose of antianxiety medication in controlling anxiety. Other studies and anecdotal evidence show that meditating improves mood, focus, and sleep; boosts emotional control; and reduces blood pressure and the release of stress hormones. According to Boston clinical psychologist Nicole Claudia, "This one practice is my favorite go-to for emotion regulation and stress reduction. It actually strengthens the pathways in the brain that allow for a more positive mood and gives you a robust tool for witnessing difficult thoughts and emotions."[12]

Meditation is an ancient practice that combines deep breathing with focusing your attention on one thing only. To meditate, individuals typically sit in a comfortable position, close their eyes, relax their muscles, and breathe in a deep, slow, natural rhythm. They focus their attention on their breath, ignoring their thoughts and whatever is happening around them. Since the mind tends to wander, this takes practice. To get back on track, if your mind wanders and thoughts drift through, one way to detach yourself from your thoughts and redirect your focus back to your breath is to envision your thoughts as balloons or clouds floating by.

There are many varieties of meditation and meditation techniques. Mantra-based meditation is one variety. A mantra is a sound, word, or phrase that you repeat in your head while you meditate to help you stay focused. Your mantra can have special meaning for you, or it can be meaningless. Some individuals find that writing their mantra down on a slip of paper that they carry around with them reminds them to calm down whenever they feel anxious.

Loving-kindness meditation is another form of meditation. Since anxious thoughts can cause you to be critical of yourself, this type of meditation helps you shift your mindset and be kinder to yourself. During loving-kindness meditation, as you breathe, you silently repeat statements, also known as affirmations, that focus on your value, such as "I am good. I am healthy. I am loved."

Meditation is most effective when it is practiced every day. Meditation websites, apps, and classes can help you learn the basics. Starting with a goal of five minutes a session is a reasonable first step. Over time, you should be able to build up to longer sessions. Adding aromatherapy by lighting scented candles infused with essential oils extracted from plants such as lavender, chamomile, bergamot, or sandalwood can enhance the relaxing effect of the session. These chemicals are known to have a calming influence on the body. So can adding soft, soothing background music or relaxing nature sounds.

It takes practice to become adept at meditating, but those who master it insist that it is well worth the effort. Music legend and founding member of the Beatles Paul McCartney is among these individuals. He says, "In moments of madness, meditation has helped me find moments of serenity—and I would like to think that it would help provide young people a quiet haven in a not-so-quiet world. . . . It is a lifelong gift, something you can call on at any time."[13]

> "In moments of madness, meditation has helped me find moments of serenity—and I would like to think that it would help provide young people a quiet haven in a not-so-quiet world."[13]
>
> —Paul McCartney, musician and founding member of the Beatles

Balancing the Mind and Body

Practicing yoga and tai chi are other relaxation strategies that have been shown to reduce anxiety and improve overall health. Both are ancient Asian disciplines that combine gentle, low-intensity stretching movements and postures with conscious breathing, mental focus, and often, meditation. Tai chi, which originated as a Chinese martial art form, involves slow dance-like movements that flow into each other. Yoga consists of specific poses and movements that build strength and flexibility as well as calming and focusing the mind. Both disciplines focus on connecting the mind and body. The goal is building balance and harmony between the two. While performing yoga and tai chi movements, you learn to detach from your thoughts and shift your attention inward, concentrating on your movements, your body positions, the muscles being used, and your breathing. In fact, yoga and tai chi practitioners coordinate their breathing with their movements. Practitioners slowly inhale as they perform expanding movements, such as raising their arms overhead. They exhale as they do contracting movements, such as twisting, bending, or lowering their arms. In addition, in many forms of yoga, practitioners hold poses for a specific number of breaths, which slows and deepens their breathing. Indeed, it is not uncommon for individuals to practice specific yoga and tai chi breathing exercises as part of their yoga and tai chi sessions. Some yoga practitioners also add meditation to their sessions.

Research has shown that both disciplines are powerful tools in managing anxiety. Both turn off the fight-or-flight response and stimulate the release of hormones that quiet the mind and calm the body. In addition, practicing yoga and tai chi raises levels of gamma-aminobutyric acid (GABA). This is a neurotransmitter, or brain chemical, that blocks the brain from sending stress- and anxiety-related messages to the body. Interestingly, research suggests that people with depression and anxiety disorders have lower-than-normal levels of GABA. In fact, some medications that

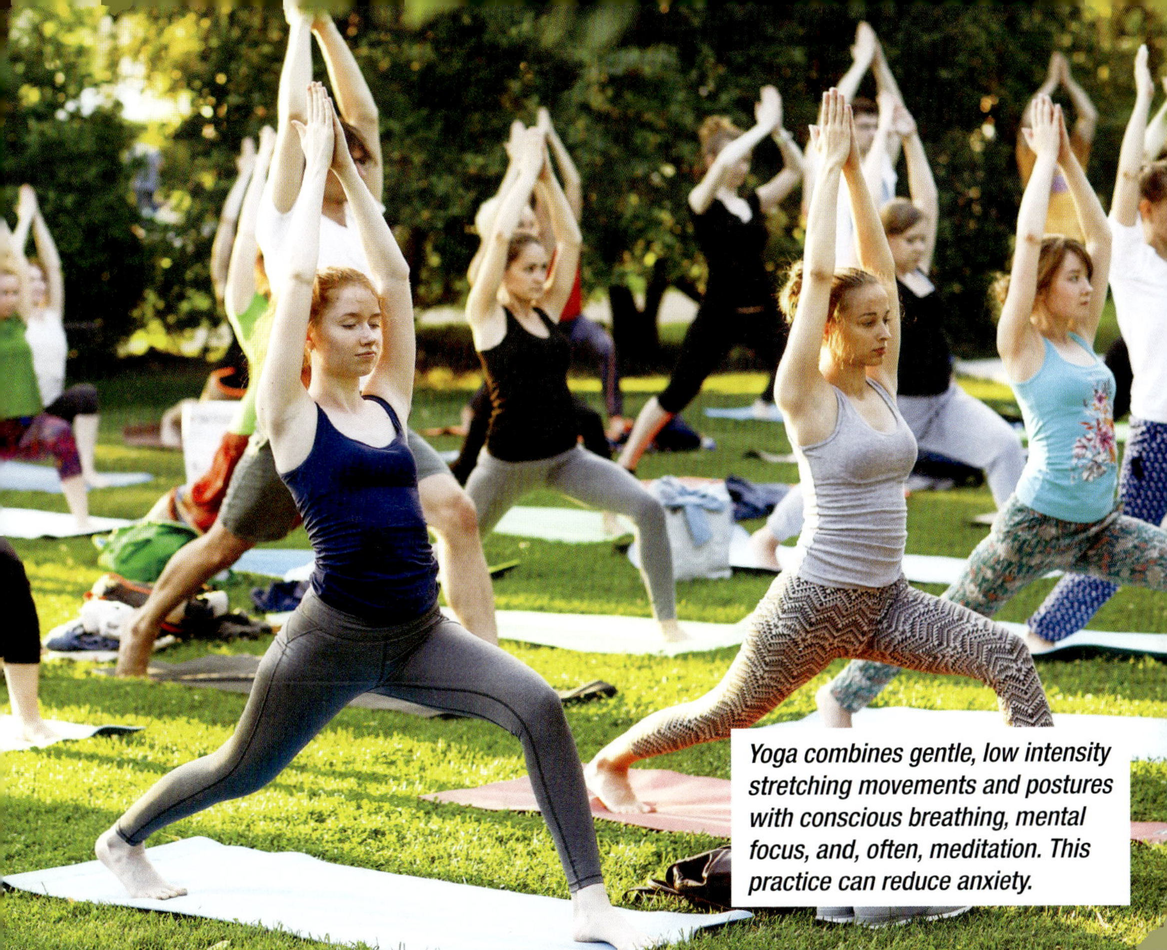

Yoga combines gentle, low intensity stretching movements and postures with conscious breathing, mental focus, and, often, meditation. This practice can reduce anxiety.

are used to treat these disorders work by raising GABA levels. Therefore, it is not surprising that many people find that practicing yoga or tai chi is a very effective weapon in battling anxiety. Michelle Lyman is one of these individuals. She is a blogger and yoga instructor who has struggled with anxiety for most of her life. Practicing yoga has helped her cope. She explains:

> I took my first yoga class and fell in love. This incredible "exercise" was more than just moving my body and breaking a sweat. I didn't know it at the time, but yoga would change my life. Over the past 22 years, I have learned movement, breathing and meditation techniques that have taught me how to stay present, recognize my anxious thoughts as just thoughts, and discover who I truly am.[14]

Living Mindfully

Living mindfully is still another strategy for quelling anxiety. When people are mindful, they focus all their attention on the present moment without worrying about the future or past—and without judging their feelings and thoughts. They accomplish this by concentrating on their surroundings—what they see, hear, smell, feel, or taste—or whatever they are doing at the current moment. Rather than multitasking, they slow down and fully focus on one thing at a time.

Being mindful helps you gain distance and control over your thoughts, rather than being overwhelmed by them. It teaches you to stay in the present, rather than worrying about the past or future and what might or might not happen. It also helps you be more accepting of your thoughts and feelings without judging yourself for having them. As a result, you reduce the body's reaction to stress, feel calmer, and are more accepting of yourself. Thus, you can experience and enjoy life more fully.

Practicing mindfulness is simple. It may be practiced in both formal and informal ways. In fact, meditation, controlled breathing, yoga, and tai chi are all formal ways to practice mindfulness. Informal mindfulness, in contrast, entails being mindful as you perform routine activities. You can apply informal mindfulness to almost every part of your daily life and practice it anywhere. You can be mindful while brushing your teeth, getting dressed, showering, eating, cooking, walking, waiting in line, commuting, talking to a friend, and so on. The possibilities are endless.

One of the easiest ways to become more mindful is by tuning in to your five senses. For instance, while making a sandwich, concentrate on what you are doing. Focus on the shape, color, texture, and aroma of the bread and the filling. Be aware of the movement of your hands and fingers as you spread, chop, and cut. Then, when you are ready to eat, eliminate any distractions; turn off your electronic devices and concentrate on the sensations you experience as you take a bite and slowly chew and

Star Gazing

Mindfulness practices are not limited to daytime. Mindful star gazing can help lower anxiety and produce a sense of calm. According to astrophysicist, author, and yoga teacher Mark Westmoquette, looking at the night sky connects people with the universe and all living things. This creates feelings of awe, which reduces stress, while the quiet and darkness add to the calming effect.

To get started, go outside on a clear night. Sit on a lawn chair or lie down in the grass and gaze up at the sky. Focus your attention on what you see and how you feel. If your mind wanders, close your eyes and breathe slowly and deeply. Then open your eyes and redirect your attention back to the stars. "Just let your mind go and appreciate this enormous planet that's underneath us," Westmoquette advises. "You don't need to know even what a star is to realize that what you're seeing is the same as every human has ever seen, and that's amazing. . . . We can just enjoy being in the dark around the stars and what it looks like and how it feels."

Quoted in Helen Carefoot, "Star Bathing Is One Shimmery, Celestial Way to Ground Yourself with Calm and Connection," Well+Good, October 21, 2023. www.wellandgood.com.

swallow. Do not think about what you need to accomplish that day or what happened earlier. Instead, turn your attention to enjoying each bite. Continue to be mindful as you sip a beverage, focusing on the drink's aroma, color, flavor, and temperature. Notice the cup, the way it looks, its size and shape, and the way it feels in your hand.

By turning off your phone, removing your headphones, and focusing your attention on your surroundings, you can continue to be mindful while you do chores, wait for public transportation, or stand in line in the supermarket. Doing sensory awareness exercises while you go about your business can keep you focused. For example, silently identifying at least three things that you hear, three things that you see, three things that you smell, and three things that you feel helps you tune out other thoughts and stay in the moment. So does focusing on a particular color and naming everything of that color that you see. The more you focus your awareness, the more your thoughts tend to slow down.

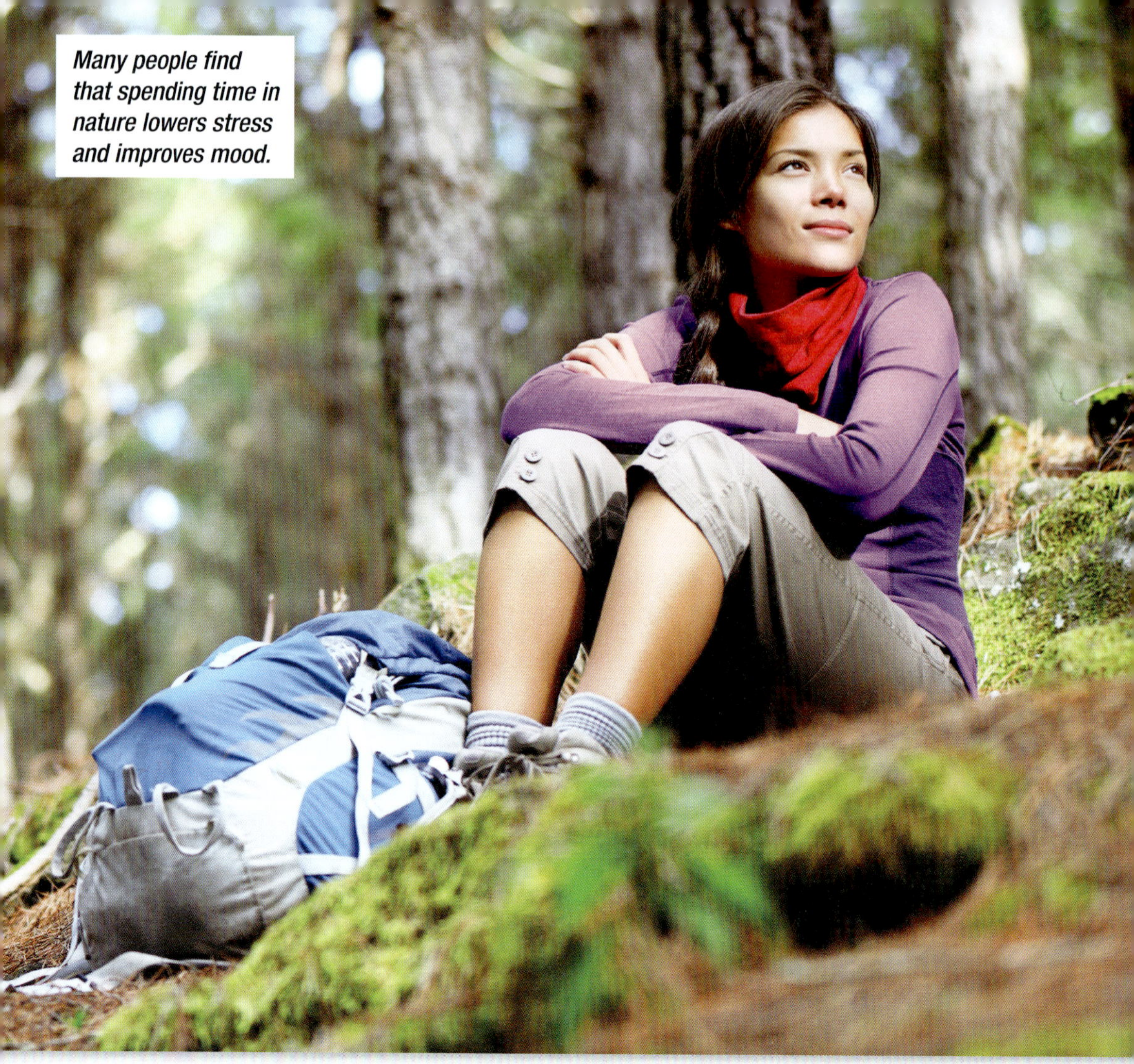

Many people find that spending time in nature lowers stress and improves mood.

To supercharge your experience, you can try applying mindfulness practice while you are outdoors. Several studies show that spending time in nature lowers stress and improves mood. According to a 2019 study published in *Frontiers in Psychology*, spending twenty to thirty minutes in nature reduces levels of the stress hormone cortisol. Therefore, combining time in nature with mindfulness practice is a powerful way to lessen anxiety. So try getting out into the fresh air, and as you walk or sit outside, notice the movement of nature. Focus on the way the sunlight shifts, the swaying of trees, the rustling of leaves, and the movement of clouds overhead.

Finding a Sense of Well-Being

You do not have to travel to an exotic location to reap the benefits of being mindful in nature. Practicing mindfulness in your own backyard can produce a sense of calm. But no matter where or when you practice mindfulness or whether the practice is formal, informal, or a combination of both, the results can help transform your mindset and improve your sense of well-being. Moreover, mindfulness practice can be especially useful during turbulent times, when we are bombarded by stressors. Indeed, a study conducted with nurses during the COVID-19 pandemic found that mindfulness training helped the subjects release tension and manage work-related stress. So when anxious thoughts fill your mind, take control by focusing on the present moment. As Canadian writer, yoga instructor, and mindfulness expert Ashley Fletcher advises, "Feel the texture of an object, listen closely to your surroundings, or focus on your breath. These techniques anchor you to reality, providing immediate calm."[15]

"Feel the texture of an object, listen closely to your surroundings, or focus on your breath. These techniques anchor you to reality, providing immediate calm."[15]

—Ashley Fletcher, writer, yoga instructor, and mindfulness expert

CHAPTER THREE

Countering Anxiety with Healthy Habits

Illustrator, writer, and entrepreneur Alex Mathers has battled anxiety for most of his life. He has tried many different strategies to help manage the condition. He found that changing his diet—more specifically, reducing his consumption of foods and beverages high in sugar and caffeine—yielded the best results. He explains:

> I'd struggled with anxiety for a large chunk of my life, but it wasn't until I made specific dietary changes that I saw a notable deduction in my experience of anxiety physically. . . . We're more depressed and anxious than ever, yet we still fill ourselves with socially acceptable drugs and stimulants [found in some foods and beverages] that worsen our anxiety. If you struggle with anxiety, much of it can be addressed via dietary changes. . . . I may get a [sugar] high from a jam donut, but think of the feeling of calm, increased performance, and self-satisfaction I gain when I can say no.[16]

Eating for Mental Health

It is not surprising that Mathers's dietary changes reduced his anxiety. The mind and body are connected. The food you eat powers you and affects both your physical and mental health.

Eating a nutrient-rich diet is an important tool in battling anxiety. According to Texas dietitian Kaleigh McMordie:

> There is evidence that diet affects mood, including depression and anxiety, as well as our body's stress response. Mood is regulated by the brain, and to work properly, the brain needs optimal fuel from nutrients in food. . . . Mood is also affected by the microbiome in the digestive tract (or the gut). [This] is why we're seeing even more emphasis on gut health in relation to mental health. Nutrient deficiencies and inflammation can be contributors to anxiety and stress, and what we eat can help or hurt these areas.[17]

Indeed, a diet rich in protein, complex carbohydrates, fiber, healthy fats, and vitamins and minerals supports overall well-being. Protein—which is found in meat, fish, seafood, poultry, eggs, milk, beans, nuts, and seeds—contains amino acids that form the basis of feel-good chemicals like serotonin and dopamine that promote relaxation and calm. Protein also builds and repairs muscles and cells, helps maintain energy, and is essential for healthy brain functioning. Oily fish in particular—such as salmon, tuna, and cod—have been found to boost brain function and reduce anxiety and depression. The oils in these fish also lessen inflammation, which is linked to multiple health issues, including anxiety and depression. Oily fish are rich in omega-3 fatty acids. Omega-3 fatty acids are healthy fats that relax muscles and reduce the production of cortisol. Pumpkin seeds, nuts, soybeans, and avocados are also chock full of omega-3 fatty acids. Pumpkin seeds are also rich in zinc, a mineral needed for the production of GABA and serotonin, feel-good chemicals that

"I'd struggled with anxiety for a large chunk of my life, but it wasn't until I made specific dietary changes that I saw a notable deduction in my experience of anxiety."[16]

—Alex Mathers, writer, illustrator, and entrepreneur

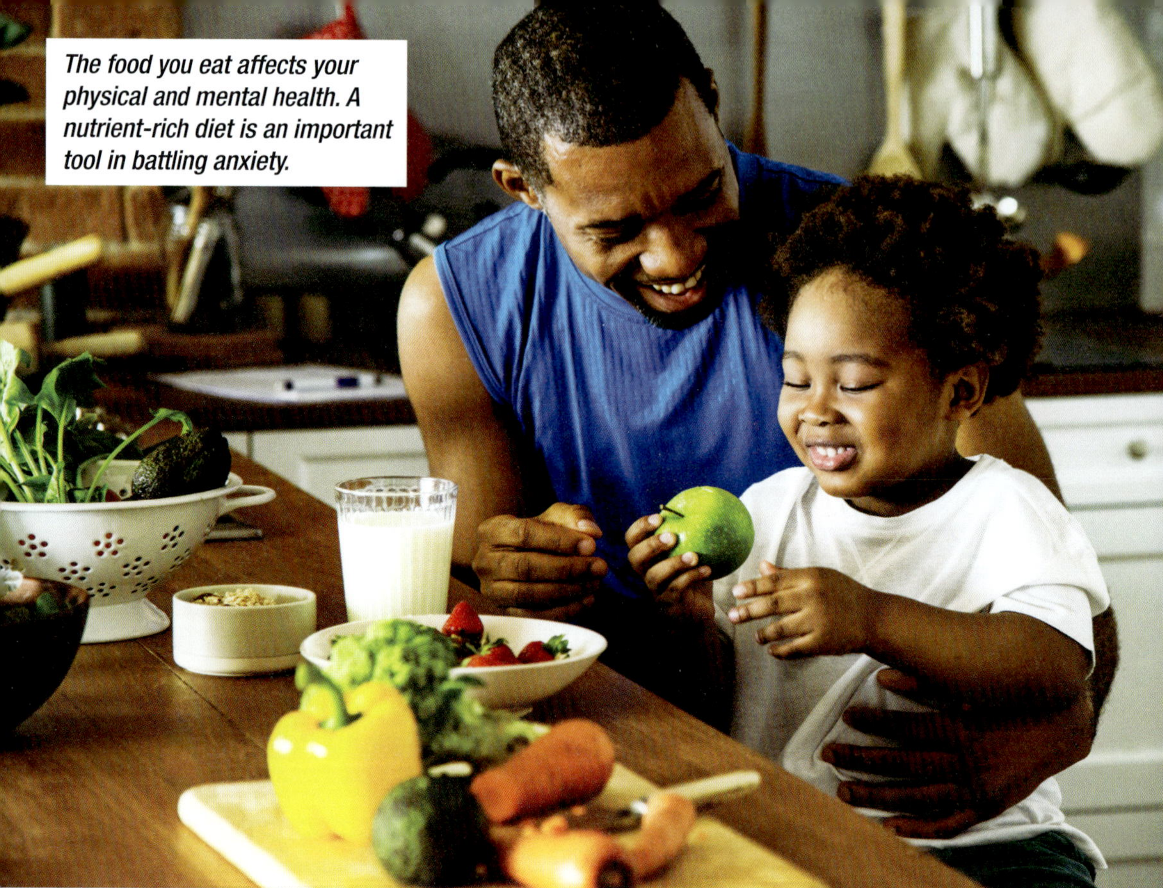

The food you eat affects your physical and mental health. A nutrient-rich diet is an important tool in battling anxiety.

relieve anxiety symptoms. Liver, beef, egg yolks, and cashew nuts are other good sources of zinc.

Other vitamins and minerals that help combat anxiety and reduce inflammation can be found in most fruits and vegetables. For example, bananas, cantaloupes, potatoes, yams, avocados, spinach, and broccoli contain potassium and magnesium, minerals that have been shown to have a calming effect on the body. Research suggests that the nutrients in bananas can relax muscles, improve sleep, lessen symptoms of depression, and boost overall mood. Writer and entrepreneur Sarah Lempa says that eating a banana whenever she is on the verge of a panic attack helps her relax. She explains:

> Despite having more run-ins with anxiety than I care to recount, I've always been determined to move through it naturally, even if that's meant trying weird things like keep-

> ing a banana in my bag 24/7. . . . But much to my surprise, it worked wonders. Minutes after I demolished the aforementioned banana . . . I felt my shoulders relax. I reveled in a much-needed deep breath. It was like waking up from a bad dream.[18]

Fruits and vegetables also contain fiber, as do beans and complex carbohydrates such as whole grain breads and cereals. Several studies point to a link between a high-fiber diet and lower risk of anxiety. Fiber helps the digestive system work efficiently, thereby improving digestive problems that can be caused by or exacerbated by anxiety. Foods that contain beneficial bacteria and yeasts, known as probiotics, also help improve digestive issues. Moreover, probiotics appear to reduce the production of cortisol and encourage the release of chemicals like serotonin that positively affect mood. Probiotics are found in fermented foods such as yogurt, sauerkraut, pickles, kimchi, tempeh, and some cheeses.

Healthy Beverages

What you drink can also help you manage anxiety. Smoothies made with fruit, yogurt, unsweetened protein powder, and dairy milk or plant milk, for example, are loaded with nutrients that help control anxiety and keep you healthy. Milk and unsweetened soy and nut milks are nutrient rich. In addition to containing vitamins and minerals, milk is an excellent source of tryptophan and melatonin, chemicals that encourage calm and help you sleep. Drinking plenty of water, too, is an important tool in managing anxiety. The body and brain need water to function well. Several studies have found that low water intake is connected to increased tension and nervousness. A 2024 Spanish study found that university students who were poorly hydrated felt the most anxious. In fact, the symptoms of dehydration mimic those of anxiety. Both conditions increase cortisol levels in the body and stimulate the release of other stress chemicals that negatively impact mood.

The Benefits of Drinking Green Tea

Despite containing a small amount of caffeine, green tea has been found to reduce anxiety and feelings of fatigue without causing the negative side effects associated with caffeine. Green tea contains L-theanine, a beneficial plant compound. Research suggests that L-theanine improves brain function, inhibits the release of stress hormones, and produces a relaxing effect on the brain and body, thereby promoting a calm, alert state.

Green tea also provides other important health benefits. It contains antioxidants. These are compounds that inhibit oxidation, a process that makes the body vulnerable to disease. Several studies have found that people who drink green tea are less likely to be diagnosed with cancer than people who do not drink green tea. Other research suggests that drinking green tea may lower the risk of developing type 2 diabetes and heart disease, as well as helping some people maintain a healthy weight.

Nonetheless, it is best not to drink green tea at bedtime, since even a small amount of caffeine can disrupt sleep. But drinking a cup or two during the day instead of coffee, sodas, energy drinks, or black tea, which contains higher levels of caffeine, may be a healthy way to battle anxiety.

To gain more control over her chronic anxiety, blogger Rizza Bermio-Gonzalez investigated how her water intake affected her anxiety symptoms. Here is what she found out: "I notice that, if I am dehydrated, my mood is affected and any symptoms of anxiety that I might normally be experiencing are exacerbated. For example, I notice that if I am dehydrated, I will experience more frequent and intense heart palpitations."[19]

Experts recommend that people drink at least five 8-ounce (237ml) glasses of water each day. If you do not like the flavor of water, you can try drinking seltzer or other unsweetened bubbly water. Or you can add a squeeze of lemon, a few berries, or a sprig of mint to your drink to enhance the taste.

Foods to Avoid or Limit

Just as certain beverages and foods can reduce anxiety, other foods and drinks can worsen the condition. Consuming highly processed, sugary, and caffeinated foods and beverages does more harm than good. Processed foods are low in essential nutrients but high in artificial ingredients, chemical additives, unhealthy fats, salt, and sugar. A diet high in processed food has been found to negatively impact mood and gut health, lead to vitamin and mineral deficiencies, and increase inflammation, all of which can contribute to feelings of anxiety. Processed meat and cheese, chips, pastries, candy, white bread, and most fast-food meals are examples of processed foods.

Sugar is a main ingredient in many processed foods, as well as in sodas and energy drinks. In fact, a 12-ounce (355 ml) can of cola contains about nine teaspoons of sugar and has no nutritional value. Consuming large amounts of sugar raises your blood sugar levels, giving you a temporary burst of energy. However, once the effect wears off, your blood sugar level plummets, causing the release of stress hormones and making you feel anxious and irritable. Kaleigh McMordie explains, "It's like a roller coaster ride for your mood. When blood sugar is dysregulated, your body will eventually kick off adrenaline, and now you are in fight-or-flight mode, which is your anxious brain. . . . A high sugar diet will dysregulate your blood sugar and contribute to stress and anxiety."[20]

Making matters worse, many sodas and almost all energy drinks contain caffeine, as do coffee, espresso, some teas, chocolate, and even some chewing gums. Caffeine is a drug that acts as a stimulant. Even small amounts can trigger the fight-or-flight response, causing physiological symptoms akin to those of anxiety. Caffeine can leave you feeling agitated and can spark a panic attack. It also interferes with sleep. And when its effects wear off, most individuals feel tired and anxious. Moreover, as with many drugs, caffeine causes dependence and withdrawal symptoms. Adding sugar to caffeinated foods and beverages only worsens the negative effects.

> "A high sugar diet will dysregulate your blood sugar and contribute to stress and anxiety."[20]
>
> —Kaleigh McMordie, dietitian

Nevertheless, it is not easy to change diet. For many people, the process of making that change adds to anxiety. Therefore, experts advise starting small by substituting a few healthy foods and drinks for ones that raise anxiety. Substituting a calming herbal tea, such as chamomile, for coffee, eating a piece of fruit rather than a donut or a candy bar, or choosing whole grain bread instead of white bread, for example, are a few positive ways to start.

Sleep Is Vital

Getting adequate sleep is also vital for good physical and mental health. While you sleep, your body performs a range of tasks that help you look and feel good and stay emotionally balanced when you awaken. Adults need seven hours of quality sleep each night, and teens need eight to ten hours. Nonetheless, millions of Americans, including one in three teenagers, do not get enough sleep. Living overscheduled, hectic lives is one reason so many people are sleep deprived. So is the stress, worry, and anxiety that are part of twenty-first-century living. Research suggests that sleep problems and anxiety are linked. The American Sleep Apnea Association reports that more than half of all insomnia cases are related to anxiety, depression, or emotional stress. This is not unexpected, since stress, worry, and anxiety make it difficult to fall asleep and stay asleep, while insufficient sleep can lead to the onset of anxiety or worsen existing anxiety. The result is a seemingly endless cycle. John Zimmer, cofounder of Lyft, experienced this cycle when his anxiety and depression were at their worst. "You get stuck in this dark cloud, and this exhaustion and this cycling of bad thoughts," he says. "[They] are compounded by the lack of sleep. Then you can't get to sleep, and things just start getting worse and worse. . . . I could not slow the negative thoughts down."[21]

Practicing healthy sleep habits can help disrupt the cycle. Keeping a consistent bedtime and wake-up time is one of these habits. It helps your brain know when it is time to go to sleep and when it is time to be alert. What you do prior to going to bed is also important. Activities that help you unwind—like taking a warm bath or shower, meditating, praying, listening to soft music, or drinking a cup of soothing warm milk or chamomile tea—help

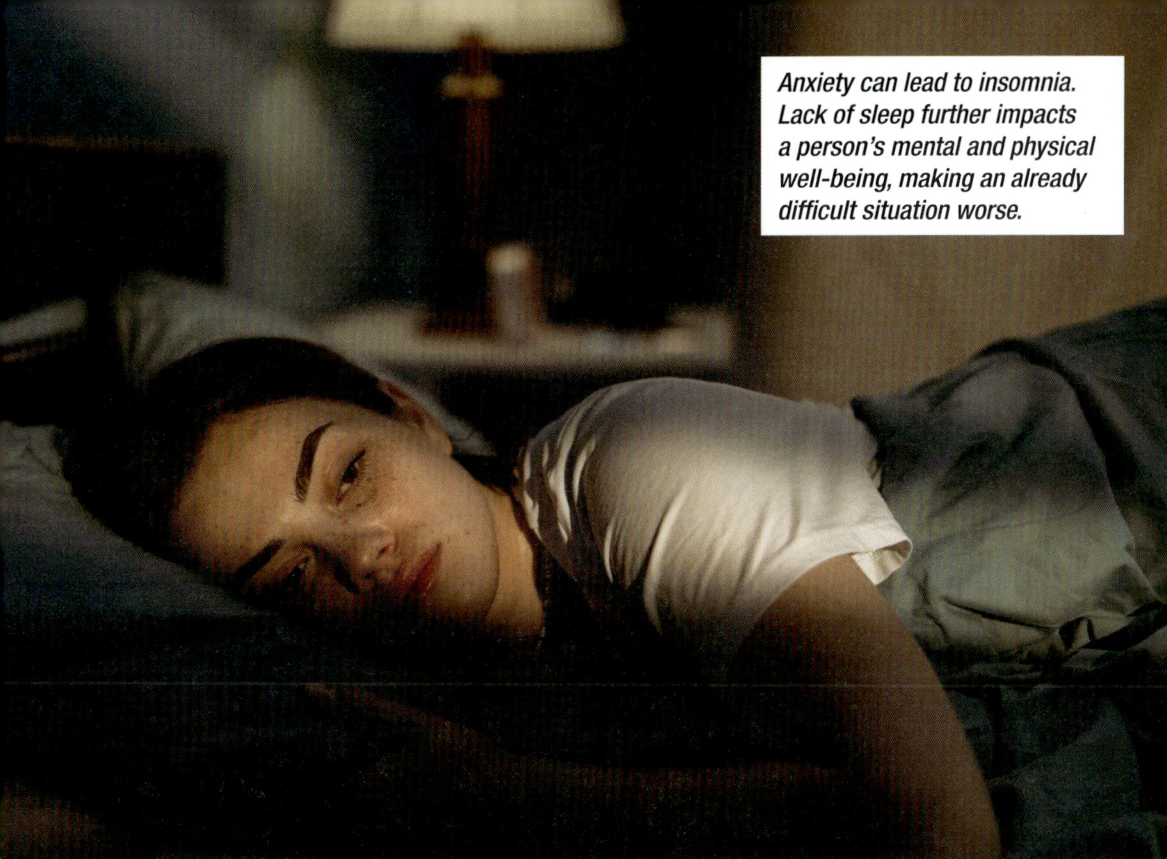

Anxiety can lead to insomnia. Lack of sleep further impacts a person's mental and physical well-being, making an already difficult situation worse.

prepare your body for sleep. Conversely, pursuing stimulating or stressful activities—such as watching the news or a disturbing movie, spending time on social media, eating a heavy meal, or consuming caffeine before going to bed—can make it difficult to get to sleep; so can the use of electronic devices before bedtime. Cell phones, video gaming devices, tablets, and computers emit a blue light that suppresses the production of melatonin, a hormone that helps you fall asleep.

Your sleep environment, too, impacts how well you sleep. Sleep experts suggest sleeping in a dark, cool, quiet room. Some individuals find that sleeping under a weighted blanket lowers their anxiety and helps them sleep better. The weight provides a deep pressure touch like that of a hug or massage, which helps you relax. The effect has been shown to reduce the release of stress hormones while increasing the release of feel-good hormones. And if you still have trouble sleeping, lying still and taking a few deep breaths can help derail anxious thoughts that keep you awake.

Dancing Anxiety Away

Dancing is a fun way to counter anxiety. Various studies have found that dancing improves brain function and mood, decreases anxious thoughts, and promotes feelings of happiness. For example, a University of California, Los Angeles, survey of one thousand dancers who battle anxiety and/or depression found that 98 percent of the respondents said that doing unchoreographed, free-flowing dance movements improved their mood. Many said it also increased their self-confidence. Another study found that participating in synchronized dance with others, such as in a Zumba class, helped people feel closer to others and form friendships.

Like other forms of exercise, dancing increases the production of endorphins, creating a feeling of general well-being. It also has a positive effect on physical health. It improves strength, flexibility, posture, and coordination, and it decreases the risk of heart disease.

Moreover, dancing does not require special equipment or even a partner. Individuals can dance alone, in groups, and with friends. They can attend virtual or in-person dance classes or hone their skills using dance video games.

Get Physical

Exercise is great for your overall health. It helps you manage your weight; strengthens your bones, heart, lungs, muscles, circulation, and immune system; and curbs anxiety. When your anxiety is raging, exercise and other physical activity can rid your body of stress chemicals. At the same time, exercise causes your body to produce and release endorphins, natural mood-boosting chemicals that produce a sense of well-being and reduce feelings of pain. Exercising also relieves stress and anxiety by diverting your attention away from your anxious thoughts and feelings and decreasing muscle tension. Plus, exercise builds self-confidence and self-esteem, which gives you a sense of control over critical thoughts. As health writer and spinning and Pilates instructor Stacey Colino testifies, "I can see the difference in my participants after each workout. They routinely leave the studio in a more upbeat mood, looking and feeling more relaxed. But it's not just them—I personally get the same benefits. Pilates and spinning regularly help me blow off steam, as well as make me feel strong and empowered."[22]

> "I can see the difference in my participants after each workout. They routinely leave the studio in a more upbeat mood, looking and feeling more relaxed."[22]
>
> —Stacey Colino, spinning and Pilates instructor

Indeed, a 2023 study published in the *British Journal of Sports Medicine* examined more than two hundred studies on the connection between exercise and mental health. The researchers found that regular exercise and physical activity can lessen psychological distress and improve symptoms of anxiety and depression. To get maximum benefits, the US government recommends that adults get a minimum of 150 minutes of moderate exercise per week and that teenagers get an hour of exercise daily or a minimum of 30 minutes three times a week.

Any form of exercise reduces anxiety, but research indicates that some activities are especially beneficial. These include walking, running or jogging, rock climbing, swimming, dancing, martial

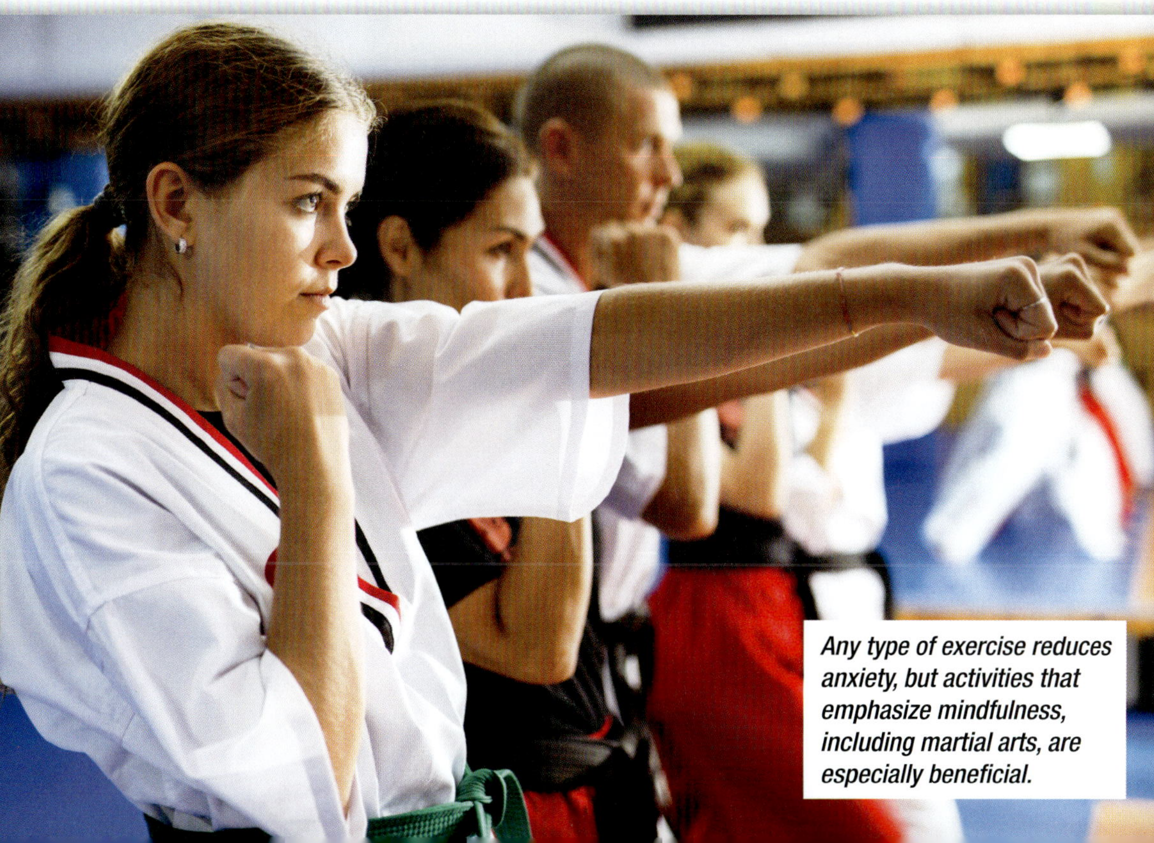

Any type of exercise reduces anxiety, but activities that emphasize mindfulness, including martial arts, are especially beneficial.

arts, and resistance training. Besides providing all the benefits of physical activity, these activities promote mindfulness. Rock climbing, for example, is "deeply meditative," according to rock climber and professional adventurer L. Renee Blount, who praises the activity for helping her manage stress. "It really helps give this deep mental break, because you're focusing on doing this one thing."[23]

Swimming offers similar mindfulness benefits. "The rhythmic nature can have a hypnotic effect, helping you get into a bit of a trance-like state,"[24] says Thomas Plante, a professor of psychology at Santa Clara University. In addition, research suggests that being in or around water is soothing. In fact, researchers at the University of Exeter in England found that even watching a video of the ocean while pedaling a stationary bike improves people's mood.

Indeed, doing any form of exercise outdoors in nature triggers a sense of calm. Walking, jogging, or running on scenic trails is a great way to relieve anxiety. Sharing the trail with a canine friend appears to provide even more benefits. Dogs can cheer you up and provide social support. But no matter where you exercise, what you do, or whether you exercise alone or with a companion, making time for physical activity is vital. Even walking for ten minutes has been shown to reduce anxiety. Adding physical activity to your daily life by taking the stairs instead of an elevator or walking instead of driving can improve your overall wellness. So can doing routine tasks and activities in which you are on your feet and moving, such as cleaning house, gardening, shoveling snow, or playing catch or frisbee with a human or canine friend. Indeed, maintaining healthy habits is a proven way to relieve anxiety and boost your physical and emotional well-being.

CHAPTER FOUR

Disconnect to Connect

Emily is a young teenager who spends most of her free time on social media. According to her parents, the more time she devotes to social media, the more anxious and sad she becomes. Out of concern for her mental health, Emily's parents unsuccessfully tried limiting her online access. Faced with this prospect, Emily threatened suicide. "It feels like the only way to remove social media and the smartphone from her life is to move to a deserted island," Emily's mother says. "She attended summer camp for six weeks each summer where no phones were permitted—no electronics at all. When we picked her up from camp she was her normal self. But as soon as she started using her phone again it was back to the same agitation and glumness."[25]

Limiting Screen Time

Technology is an integral part of twenty-first-century daily life. The availability of smartphones allows individuals to be online around the clock. In fact, 46 percent of teen and 62 percent of young adult respondents to a Pew Research Center survey released in 2024 said that they are online almost constantly. Many of these individuals admitted to experiencing FOMO, or fear of missing out on events occurring on social media when they disconnect. FOMO triggers anxiety in many social media users, causing them to compulsively check their

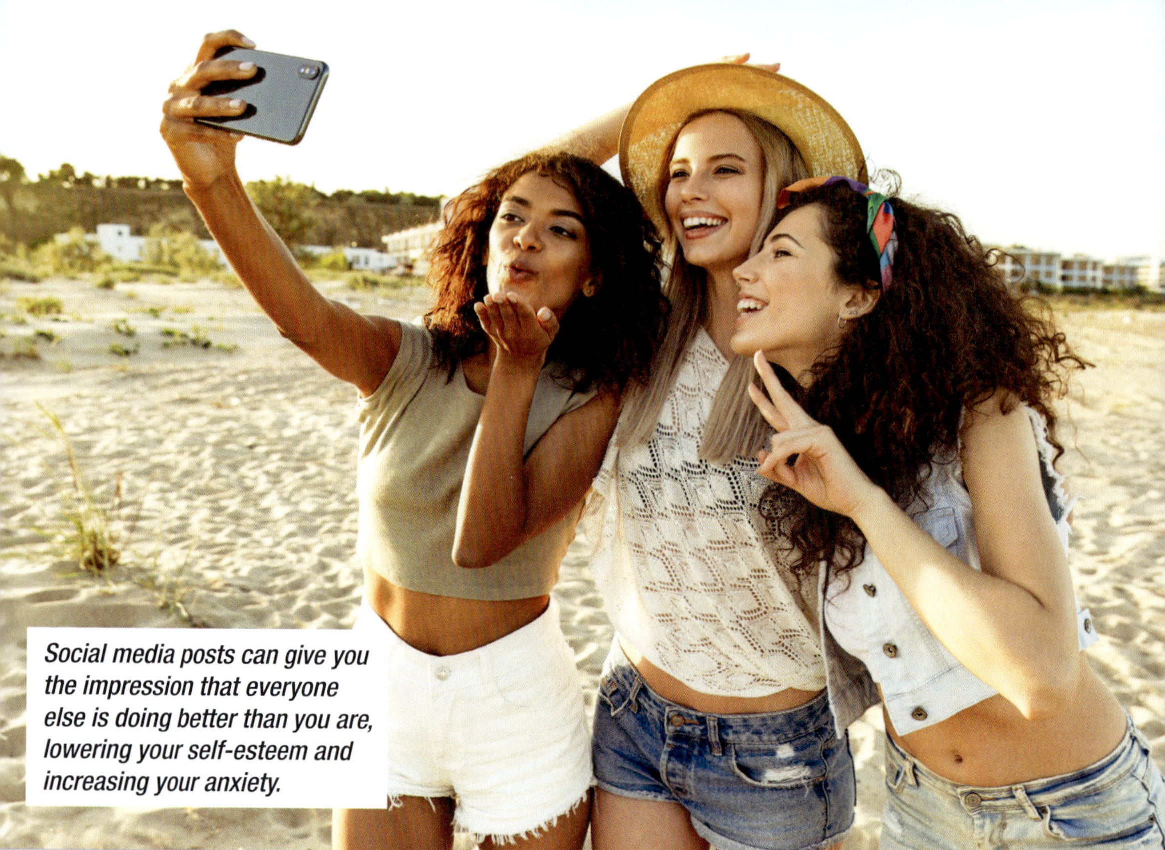

Social media posts can give you the impression that everyone else is doing better than you are, lowering your self-esteem and increasing your anxiety.

phones. This preoccupation with social media can negatively interfere with sleep and distract you from school or work obligations, personal projects, and relationships, which can add to anxiety.

In 2024 the online news site Politico surveyed fourteen hundred mental health professionals about the causes of the current mental health crisis in the United States. More than one-quarter blamed social media use. Research indicates that anxiety and social media use are closely related. A 2022 study from the University of Auckland in New Zealand, for example, divided a group of college students into two groups. Those in one group took a weeklong break from social media, while those in the other continued their regular use. The group that took a break experienced a significant reduction in feelings of stress and depression, while the other group reported no change in emotional state.

One reason why engaging with social media can jump-start anxiety is that many social media users post only the most exciting, most flattering, and most eye-catching details about their lives. Viewing these posts can leave people feeling as though nothing in their own lives can ever measure up. This experience can produce feelings of envy, lower self-esteem, and boost anxiety. Plus, those who use social media without strong privacy settings open themselves up to negative and hurtful comments that can trigger or worsen anxiety. Negative interactions in texts, emails, and chat rooms have a similar effect.

Not even celebrities are immune from negativity on social media. Actress and singer Selena Gomez, for example, was so troubled by some of the mean comments her social media platform was receiving that she stopped using social media for a while. She explains, "I have problems with depression and anxiety. . . . At one point Instagram became my whole world, and it was really dangerous. . . . Taking a break from social media was the best decision that I've ever made for my mental health. . . . The unnecessary hate . . . went away once I put my phone down."[26]

Indeed, taking a break from or putting time limits on your social media usage can help lessen anxiety, but FOMO can make this difficult to do. Nevertheless, it is not necessary to swear off social media entirely to reap the benefits. Even cutting back by one hour per week can help. As you become more comfortable disconnecting, you can try building up to one hour a day, then slowly increase the time. To help you maintain your commitment, try not to look at your phone while you are eating, exercising, driving, or interacting with others in real time. Selecting specific times for checking and responding to online messages and notifications can make the process easier, but if the pull is too great, try turning your phone off when you are doing other things.

> **"I have problems with depression and anxiety. . . . At one point Instagram became my whole world, and it was really dangerous. . . . Taking a break from social media was the best decision that I've ever made for my mental health."[26]**
>
> —Selena Gomez, actress and singer

Connecting to Creative Activities

Spending less time online gives you more time to devote to creative pursuits. Extensive research indicates that daily participation in a creative activity can significantly reduce a person's anxiety level, improve mood, and increase feelings of happiness and general well-being. When you are engaged in a creative activity, you are practicing mindfulness. In fact, being fully focused on a creative project affects the mind and body in the same way as meditation. It inhibits the release of stress hormones and promotes the release of feel-good chemicals that calm and relax you. Moreover, participating in a creative activity provides you with an emotional outlet to express feelings that may be difficult for you to express in other ways. That is the case for Tim Bernard, a young man who writes and plays music to battle anxiety and depression. He explains, "I can honestly say that without the outlet of music, I would be in a much darker place than I am today. I've managed to pour the emotion, fear, and hopelessness of my mental struggles into my music. . . . It's become a cathar-

Music and the Mind

Making and listening to music are creative hobbies that help battle anxiety. Singing, for instance, raises oxytocin levels. Oxytocin is a feel-good chemical that has a calming effect on the body. It improves mood and promotes the formation of social connections. Indeed, research suggests that singing and harmonizing with others creates a bond between singers.

Listening to music can also lessen anxiety by relaxing you. In fact, several studies have found that when people are being prepped for surgery, if they listen to soothing music, they have lower blood pressure and heart rate and require less pain medication than people who do not listen to music before surgery. Listening to music also affects mood. It appears that the best music to lower stress and anxiety is music with a tempo of sixty beats per minute. This tempo is believed to raise alpha brain waves linked to a calm mind. In addition to tempo, the style of the music affects a listener's mood. Listening to happy music has been found to make people feel happier, while listening to sad or angry music can have a negative effect on people who feel sad or angry.

sis for me and the most effective way to articulate how I feel and what I'm going through mentally."[27]

“To me, my creative hobbies are a way to impose order upon chaos. Anxiety generally makes me feel like my life is chaotic even when 99% of the time it isn't, so to have the ability to impose a sense of order is valuable.”[28]

—T.J. Desalvo, blogger

In addition, completing a project boosts your sense of accomplishment and self-esteem. And since you decide on every color, stitch, word, note, and so on that you use, working on a creative project gives you a sense of control, which chronic anxiety can take from you. T.J. Desalvo, a blogger who battles chronic anxiety, concurs. He says:

> To me, my creative hobbies are a way to impose order upon chaos. Anxiety generally makes me feel like my life is chaotic even when 99% of the time it isn't, so to have the ability to impose a sense of order is valuable. Writing allows me to craft art out of random words—video editing allows me to craft a narrative out of what would otherwise be a random assortment of clips. . . . I also enjoy seeing my projects slowly take shape from nothing. Also, it gives me more time to get lost in whatever I am doing, which to me is valuable in itself.[28]

Nor do you have to create a masterpiece to enjoy the benefits of creative activities. The process and the soothing way it makes you feel are just as important as the finished product. Bread making, for example, requires you to squeeze and squish dough with your hands. This action helps you release stress and tension even if the final product is not perfect. Similarly, the repetitive and rhythmic movement of knitting, crocheting, and weaving has an especially calming effect on the mind and body.

There are seemingly countless creative outlets you can try. Gardening, coloring, singing, writing, and playing an instrument are just a few possibilities. So are photography, woodworking, nail art, and building models, among many other activities. Soccer great David Beckham, for instance, builds things with LEGO bricks when he feels anxious. Moreover, you can practice your craft alone or as part of a group. Participating in a shared activity is a good way to make new friends. But whatever you choose to do, to reap the benefits, it should be something you enjoy. If you find that an activity does not suit you, do not worry about it. Try something else instead. Creative pursuits should not feel like chores. They should be fun and relaxing.

Helping Others

Helping others through volunteering and compassionate actions are other offline undertakings that aid in reducing anxiety. These actions are especially helpful in tumultuous times when the impact of seemingly endless news reports and graphic images of global threats and crises can leave you feeling powerless and fearful about the future. These feelings can trigger disturbing thoughts about issues that are beyond any one person's control. Hence, although it is important to keep up with current events, it is wise to limit the time you spend viewing troubling news. Rather than viewing a continuous loop of disturbing news, taking steps to make the world a better place empowers you. It gives you back a sense of purpose and control. And it helps you feel valued, boosting your sense of self-worth. In fact, helping others has been shown to reduce anxiety and increase hopefulness about the future. It triggers the release of oxytocin, a feel-good hormone associated with happiness.

You do not have to be a hard-core activist to reap the benefits of giving back. You can do small things that have a positive impact. For instance, if climate change and other environmental issues make you anxious, consider planting a tree, picking up litter, or joining a group that lobbies for green legislation or supports environmentally minded political candidates. Similarly, if you are troubled by the fate of vulnerable populations, you could donate to a charity that helps the poor, take part in a local food

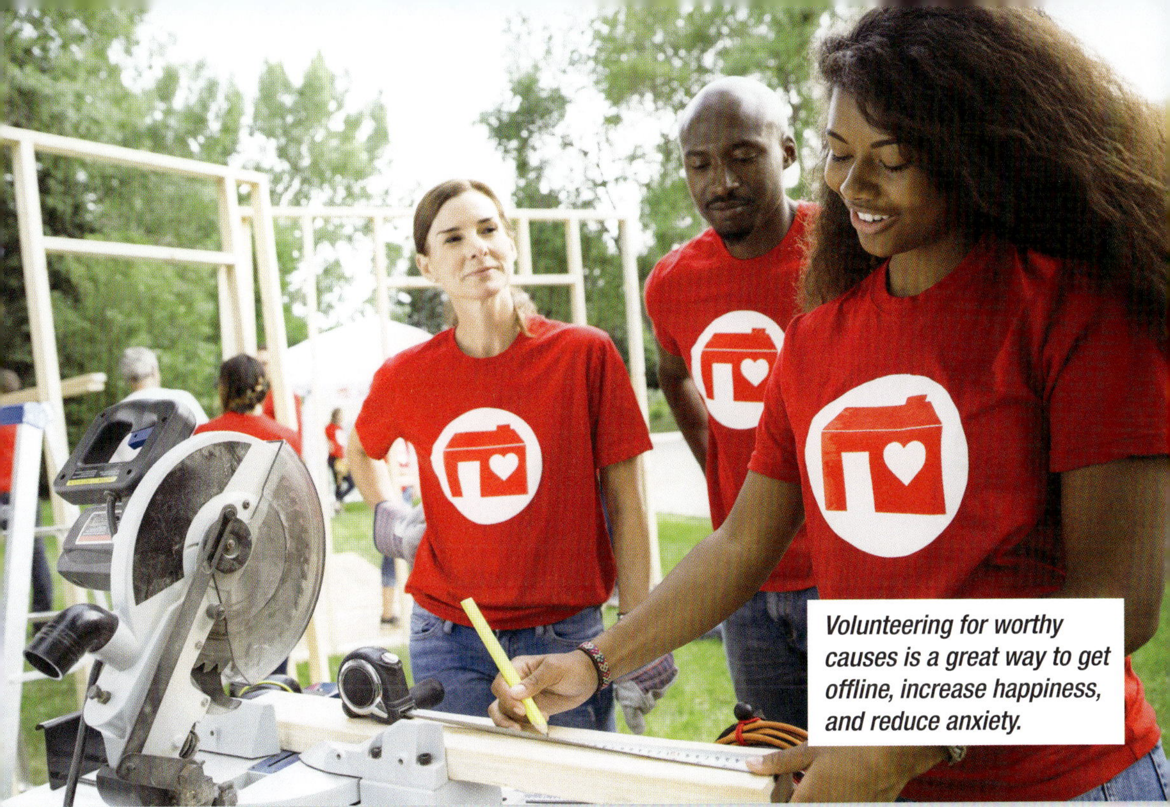

Volunteering for worthy causes is a great way to get offline, increase happiness, and reduce anxiety.

drive, or give clothes and objects you no longer use to a rescue mission. And if gun violence and global conflicts are stressing you out, joining a group dedicated to preventing violence can empower you. Lighting a candle or saying a prayer for those involved in violent conflicts, participating in a vigil, or contacting your congressperson to express your concerns are other steps you can consider.

Indeed, even small acts of kindness such as offering to cut an elderly neighbor's grass, fostering a pet, or saying a kind word to someone who is feeling down can brighten your world as well as that of others. As associate professor of psychology at the University of California, Santa Barbara, Erika Felix, explains, "Feeling like you're doing something gives you agency and control. Having purposeful action helps our mental health."[29]

> "Feeling like you're doing something gives you agency and control. Having purposeful action helps our mental health."[29]
>
> —Erika Felix, associate professor of psychology

Connecting to Supportive People

Connecting to people whom you trust also helps improve mental health. Humans are social creatures. We need positive social interaction to thrive. Although online communities can help you connect with others, multiple studies suggest that connecting virtually is not as beneficial in lowering anxiety as in-person contact. And even though chatting on the phone or texting with a loved one does provide a social connection and can help reduce stress, it appears that physical touch and eye-to-eye contact has a greater effect on calming the body. Numerous studies confirm that having good, in-person, social relationships promotes feelings of happiness. It also helps reduce feelings of isolation and loneliness that often accompany chronic anxiety. Plus, talking about your concerns and worries with a trusted friend or family member makes you feel heard and loved. It provides you with a fresh perspective, a supportive environment for managing stress, and positive emotional support.

Nevertheless, it is important to avoid unhealthy, toxic relationships. Friendships with people who tear you down, do not take your problems seriously, focus solely on themselves, or push you around can increase your stress and anxiety. It is best to avoid these individuals, or at least limit the amount of time you spend with them. Instead, look to friends and family members who genuinely care about you to provide a sympathetic ear and emotional support. And keep in mind that you, too, need to be supportive of members of your social network when they are having problems. Being there for each other helps build your connection.

Getting Professional Help

When anxiety becomes overwhelming and significantly interferes with your daily life, you may need more help and support than a friend or family member can offer. If you feel angry, frightened, worried, or depressed most of the time or have suicidal thoughts, connecting with a mental health professional can help you gain

Assertiveness and Social Connections

Anxiety can keep people from standing up for themselves. Anxious thoughts can make individuals struggle to express their needs and wants or set boundaries. Distorted thinking causes them to imagine that if they do not accede to others, they will be rejected, and bad things will happen as a result. Therefore, it is common for people with anxiety to go along with whatever others decide, even if it is contrary to their needs or beliefs. They have trouble saying no and frequently take on too many tasks or participate in activities that they would rather not take part in. As a result, they often feel resentful, victimized, ignored, and angry. These emotions can lessen self-esteem and worsen anxiety symptoms.

This type of passive behavior can also make it difficult to build and maintain good social connections. It can damage relationships and weaken mutual trust and respect. Expressing your wants and needs in a calm and respectful manner, on the other hand, improves communication and helps create mutual understanding and more harmonious relationships.

control of your life. As New York art therapist Erica Wickett explains, "When I meet with clients struggling with these issues, they've hit a breaking point where their lives feel like it no longer makes sense to them. This feeling can be incredibly isolating and often there is a need for help outside of their existing support systems to help them make sense of things again."[30]

Psychologists, psychiatrists, counselors, pastoral counselors, social workers, primary care physicians, and specialized therapists are some of the various mental health professionals who can help. Unfortunately, some individuals hesitate to seek professional help because they do not want to appear weak or dependent. Societal stigmas about anxiety and mental health disorders can make people feel ashamed of their condition. And fear of being judged causes some individuals to deny they have a problem, which can worsen anxiety symptoms. Still, despite unfair stigmas, getting professional help for a mental health issue is no different from getting medical help for a physical problem. It is not a sign of weakness or failure. By helping you identify anxiety triggers,

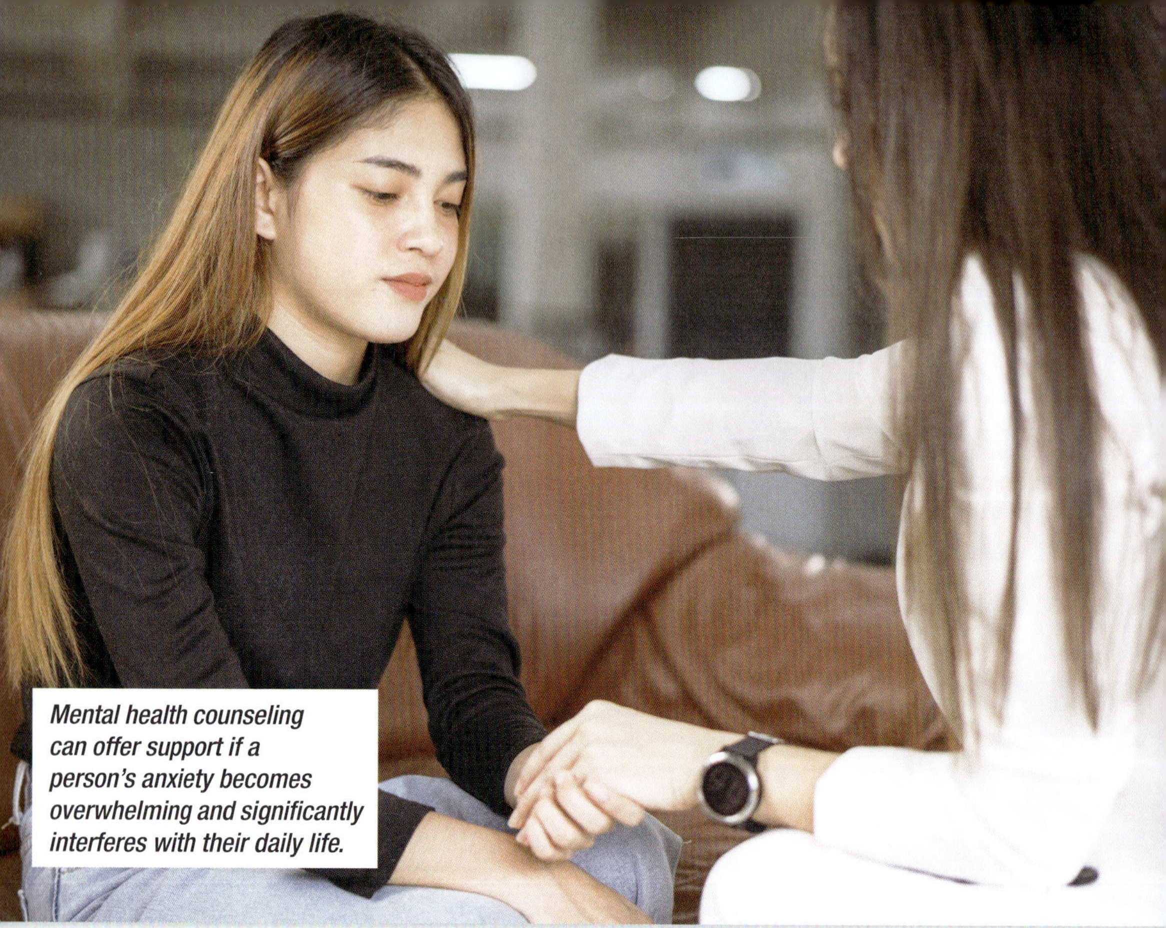

Mental health counseling can offer support if a person's anxiety becomes overwhelming and significantly interferes with their daily life.

understand anxiety symptoms, and develop coping strategies, mental health therapy can give you the tools you need to restructure the way you think so that you can face your fears.

There are several different types of mental health treatments that have proved effective in helping individuals manage anxiety. Cognitive behavioral therapy (CBT) is one of the most popular. Through talk therapy sessions, patients are helped to recognize and confront distorted thoughts and specific behaviors that trigger their anxiety. They also learn a variety of strategies to change these thoughts and behaviors. These strategies often include mindfulness practices. CBT may also include exposure therapy, a practice in which patients are gradually exposed to activities, objects, and ideas that trigger their anxiety so that they can face and manage their fears. Exposure therapy is especially helpful in managing phobias and social anxiety disorder.

Sometimes, medication is also prescribed to help manage symptoms. Only licensed physicians and nurse practitioners can prescribe medication. Several different types of medication are used, including antidepressants, tranquilizers, and beta blockers. Antidepressants such as Zoloft work by increasing serotonin levels, which helps improve mood. But they do not work right away. It takes two to six weeks for such antidepressants to take effect, and the medication is usually taken for six months to one year before it is gradually reduced. Tranquilizers like Xanax work more rapidly. Tranquilizers increase the effect of GABA, which has an immediate calming effect on the body. Tranquilizers are often taken on an as-needed basis.

When used to treat anxiety, beta blockers are also taken as needed. Beta blockers are mostly prescribed for heart-related conditions such as high blood pressure and irregular heartbeat. But because they turn off the fight-or-flight response, beta blockers also help manage the physical symptoms of anxiety like trembling, dizziness, and a rapid heartbeat.

Still, despite their benefits, like all medications, antianxiety medications can have troubling side effects, and antidepressants and tranquilizers can lead to addiction. However, when these medications are taken as prescribed, under the care of a medical professional, they can provide you with the relief you need to heal. Indeed, with all the traditional and holistic strategies that are available to help manage anxiety, there is no reason to let anxiety take charge of your life. So take a deep, calming breath and get started. Your mental health and overall well-being are worth the effort.

SOURCE NOTES

Introduction: Living in Turbulent Times

1. Daneisha Carter, "Finding the Light at the End of the Tunnel," ADAA, August 31, 2023. https://adaa.org.
2. Quoted in Calley Nelson, "16 Celebrities with Anxiety Disorders," Everyday Health, October 28, 2022. www.everydayhealth.com.
3. Quoted in Victoria Whalen, "ACE Interview: Jorge Alvarez on Mental Health Activism and Climate Change," Action for the Climate Emergency, June 24, 2022. https://acespace.org.
4. Carter, "Finding the Light at the End of the Tunnel."

Chapter One: Understanding Anxiety

5. Quoted in Allie Griffin, "Jonah Hill Will No Longer Promote His New Movies to Avoid Anxiety Attacks," *New York Post*, August 18, 2022. www.nypost.com.
6. Quoted in Fjolla Arifi, "5 Signs You're in a Constant State of 'Fight or Flight,'" Huffington Post, June 26, 2023. www.huffingtonpost.co.uk.
7. Danielle E., "My Battle and Triumph over OCD, Anxiety and Depression," National Alliance on Mental Illness, 2024. www.nami.org.
8. Quoted in Nelson, "16 Celebrities with Anxiety Disorders."
9. Quoted in Kayla Hui, "I Wrote in a Gratitude Journal for 45 Days to Lower My Stress and Improve My Sleep—Here's What Happened," Well+Good, February 14, 2023. www.wellandgood.com.

Chapter Two: Mastering Relaxation Techniques

10. Quoted in Kate Booggard, "5 Ways to Calm Your Nerves, According to Olympic Athletes," The Muse, June 19, 2020. www.themuse.com.

11. Quoted in Booggard, "5 Ways to Calm Your Nerves, According to Olympic Athletes."
12. Nicole Claudia, "A Holistic Approach to Managing Anxiety," *The Whole Truth* (blog), *Psychology Today*, June 29, 2021. www.psychologytoday.com.
13. Quoted in Prixal, "Sir Paul McCartney Received a 'Gift of Meditation,'" Meditation Lifestyle, February 20, 2024. www.meditationlifestyle.com.
14. Michelle Lyman, "My Personal Struggle with Anxiety and How to Keep Moving Forward," Serenity Yoga and Wellness, January 24, 2022. www.serenityyogawellness.com.
15. Ashley Fletcher, "Halting the Spiral: Navigating Repetitive Thought Patterns," Mindful, March 12, 2024. www.mindful.org.

Chapter Three: Countering Anxiety with Healthy Habits

16. Alex Mathers, "7 Small Dietary Shifts That Will Dramatically Reduce Your Anxiety," Your Tango, March 4, 2024. www.yourtango.com.
17. Quoted in Cathy Cassata, "The Experts Agree: What You Eat Can Directly Impact Stress and Anxiety," Verywell Mind, January 3, 2023. www.verywellmind.com.
18. Sarah Lempa, "How an Emotional Support Banana Became My Secret Weapon Against Anxiety," Well+Good, October 12, 2023. www.wellandgood.com.
19. Rizza Bermio-Gonzalez, "How Your Diet Affects Your Anxiety," HealthyPlace, August 11, 2020. www.healthyplace.com.
20. Quoted in Cassata, "The Experts Agree."
21. Quoted in Marissa Charles, "Lyft Co-Founder John Zimmer Reveals Overwhelming Stress Led to Cycling of Bad Thoughts and Depression," *People*, May 27, 2022. www.people.com.
22. Stacey Colino, "Stress Relieving Exercises That Help You Feel More Relaxed and Empowered," *U.S. News & World Report*, July 8, 2024. www.health.usnews.com.

23. Quoted in Angela Haupt, "Rock Climbing Is a Thrill. It's Also Really Good for You," *Time*, February 16, 2023. www.time.com.
24. Quoted in Colino, "Stress Relieving Exercises That Help You Feel More Relaxed and Empowered."

Chapter Four: Disconnect to Connect

25. Quoted in Jonathan Haidt, "Generation Anxiety: Smartphones Have Created a Gen Z Mental Health Crisis—but There Are Ways to Fix It," *The Guardian* (Manchester, UK), March 24, 2024. www.theguardian.com.
26. Quoted in Julie Mazziotta, "Selena Gomez 'Found It Difficult to Be Me' as She Dealt with 'Depression and Anxiety,'" *People*, January 6, 2022. www.people.com.
27. Tim Bernard and Mike Bernard, "It Sounded Better in My Head," Anxiety and Depression Association of America, September 28, 2023. www.adaa.org.
28. T.J. Desalvo, "Is Getting Lost in a Hobby Good for Your Mental Health?," HealthyPlace, February 16, 2022. www.healthyplace.com.
29. Quoted in Molly Longman, "How to Cope with Watching War Unfold, According to Mental Health Experts," *Teen Vogue*, November 14, 2023. www.teenvogue.com.
30. Quoted in Cathy Cassata, "Michael Phelps: My Depression and Anxiety Is Never Going to Just Disappear," Healthline, May 17, 2022. www.healthline.com.

Getting Help and Information

Books

Barbara Diggs, *Relax: How to Manage Anxiety and Emotions in an Uncertain World*. San Diego, CA: ReferencePoint, 2023.

Bruce Hyman et al., *More than Stress: Understanding Anxiety Disorders*. Minneapolis, MN: Twenty-First Century, 2024.

Scientific American Editors, *Navigating Anxiety and Depression*. New York: Scientific American Educational, 2023.

Katherine Speller, *The Beasts in Your Brain*. Minneapolis, MN: Zest, 2023.

Internet Sources

Daryl Austin, "What Is Mindfulness? Try This Meditation to Calm Down and Be Present," *USA Today*, April 24, 2023. www.usatoday.com.

Cathleen Crichton-Stuart and Aline Diaz, "What Are Some Foods to Ease Anxiety?," Medical News Today, January 16, 2024. www.medicalnewstoday.com.

Sharon Lee, "Methods of Calming Anxiety: The Guide," Fearless Pursuits, April 8, 2024. www.fearlesspursuits.com.

Traci Pedersen, "What Type of Psychotherapy Is Best for Anxiety?," Healthline, January 17, 2023. www.healthline.com.

Melinda Smith et al., "Anxiety Disorders and Anxiety Attacks," HelpGuide.org, July 17, 2024. www.helpguide.org.

Websites

Anxiety & Depression Association of America (ADAA)
https://adaa.org
The ADAA provides information and help to people with anxiety and depression. It offers a wealth of information about these conditions and how to manage them, personal stories written by people with these conditions, help in finding therapists and support groups, webinars, videos, blogs, and peer-to-peer online communities.

Mental Health America (MHA)
www.mhanational.org
MHA is a nonprofit organization dedicated to improving mental health. Using a peer-to-peer approach, it offers information on various mental health conditions such as anxiety and depression, mental health screening tests, treatment information, online support groups, and crisis resources.

National Alliance on Mental Illness (NAMI)
www.nami.org
The NAMI is a large mental health organization dedicated to educating, supporting, advocating for, and improving the lives of people with mental health problems and their loved ones. It offers tons of information, personal stories, links to support groups all over the United States, a helpline, podcasts, on-campus support clubs, a newsletter, reports, and resource guides.

988 Suicide & Crisis Lifeline
https://988lifeline.org
This organization provides free, confidential support by trained counselors to individuals who are considering suicide or need emotional support. Counselors can be reached by calling or texting 988. They are available twenty-four hours a day, seven days a week.

QuietKit

https://quietkit.com

This website offers information about meditation and how to meditate, instructions on different controlled deep-breathing techniques, and free guided meditation sessions for beginners.

Verywell Mind

www.verywellmind.com

Verywell Mind offers mental health information, guidance, and help on various mental health conditions, including anxiety and anxiety disorders. It provides lots of information about treatments, medication, self-care, and management techniques such as meditation, mindfulness, and controlled breathing. It also provides guided meditation videos and links to online therapy sources.

INDEX

Note: Boldface page numbers indicate illustrations.

PICTURE CREDITS

Cover: haveseen/Shutterstock

6: PeopleImages.com-Yuri A/Shutterstock
9: Fotos593/Shutterstock
13: FiledIMAGE/Shutterstock
16: PeopleImages.com-Yuri A/Shutterstock
20: Pathoc/Shutterstock
25: David Tadevosian/Shutterstock
28: MariDav/Shutterstock
32: Rawpixel.com/Shutterstock
37: Lysenko Andrey/Shutterstock
39: BearFotos/Shutterstock
42: DeanDrobat/Shutterstock
47: Hero Images Inc/Shutterstock
50: Wirestock Creators/Shutterstock

ABOUT THE AUTHOR

Barbara Sheen is the author of 115 books for young people. She lives in New Mexico with her family. In her spare time, she likes to swim, practice yoga, garden, cook, and read.